Matth

why we should

~~work harder~~

~~push to the limit~~

~~be more productive~~

[sleep]

smarter

The Scientific Blueprint to Optimize Your Energy Levels and Supercharge Your Day

Why We Should Sleep Smarter

The Scientific Blueprint to Optimize Your Energy Levels and Supercharge Your Day

Table of Contents

Introduction

Sleeping: The Unappreciated Skill *13*

Chapter 1: Four Myths About Sleep

Myth No. 1: Your Brain Rests While You Sleep..................... 18

Myth No. 2: You Need Less Sleep as You Get Older......... 21

Myth No. 3: You Can Catch Up on Sleep................................ 24

Myth No. 4: Sleep Timing Doesn't Matter.............................. *26*

Chapter 2: The Power of Slumber

Sleep and Longevity... 30

Sleep as a Reset... 32

Sleep, Memory, and Cognitive Function................................ 33

Sleep and Immune Function... 36

Sleep and Mood.. 37

How Much Sleep is Enough.. 39

Chapter 3: Mastering Your Sleep Cycle

The Circadian Rythm: Your Inner Time-Keeper.................. 42

Cortisol: Hack Your Inner Alarm Clock.................................... 44

Adenosine: The Bodys' Natural Sleep Aid............................. 46

The Yin and Yang Hormones of Sleep Regulation............ 48

How Stress Can Disrupt Our Sleep-Wake Balance........... 50

Tool 1... 52

Chapter 4: Perfect Your Morning

Make Sunlight Your Best Friend.. 56

Tool 2 57

Tool 3 58

Tool 4 60

Chapter 5: Maintain a Productive Day

Tool 5 64

Tool 6 66

Tool 7 72

Chapter 6: Fall Asleep Like a Pro

Tool 8 74

Tool 9 77

Tool 10 81

Chapter 7: How to Deal With Sleep Interruptions

The „Bathroom-Break" Type 86

Tool 11 86

The „Active-Mind" Type 87

Tool 12 88

The „Insomniac" Type 90

Chapter 8: Adaptive Strategies to Boost Your Success

Chronotypes 94

Tool 13 96

Social Jet Lag 97

Travelling Abroad 99

Shift Work 103

Parenthood 106

Supplements to Fortify Your Rest 110

Final Thoughts 115

Introduction

A third of our entire lifetime is spent sleeping. For the typical adult, this equates to about 26 years of our lives being spent asleep (Kandel et al., 2012). *Twenty-six years.* If that doesn't convince you that sleep is the most important cornerstone of our health, then I don't know what will! This estimation, however, relies on the standard suggestion that adults get eight hours of restful slumber every night. Unfortunately, this could not be farther from the truth, as the average sleep duration and quality are on a massive decline. Even though experts agree that most adults need between seven and nine hours of rest per night, a large percentage of today's population routinely gets much less (Jones, 2013).

Ironically, many adherents of the hustle-grind culture are convinced that getting eight hours of downtime each night is far too much! There is a widespread belief among today's performance-driven people that sleep is a waste of time and that those hours would be better spent "working one's nose to the grindstone."

What they may not realize is that this third of our lives is spent for the purpose of rejuvenation. That's right, our rest breaks revitalize our brains and bodies, giving us the energy we need to focus and produce high-quality work. Deep sleep improves our mental and physical capacities in a lot of different ways, from our memory to our immune system, our weight, our mood, hormones, and reproduction. So rest assured that by the end of reading this book, you'll have learned everything about how this sleep inadequacy will eventually take its toll.

Interestingly, during the COVID-19 pandemic, many people were forced to re-evaluate their priorities in this modern day and age and were drawn to take a step in the right direction with their lives.

According to the latest research, there has been an increasing shift in focus on quality of life over the decades (Roser, 2016). Perhaps that is why physical and mental well-being were all recently reported as the highest indicators of happiness around the world. Now, it seems that more and more people want to prioritize their health, and hence, the spotlight has been shone brightly on sleep as perhaps the most essential pillar.

But education on this topic can be incredibly difficult. For anyone who doesn't have the required background knowledge, it would be tricky to navigate all the intricacies of science alone, from the jargon used to how research is conducted and the way results of studies are interpreted. It is much like piecing together a puzzle without knowing what the final picture is supposed to look like.

So, how does one go about educating themselves on the core principles of sleep?

That is where this book comes in.

I'm Matthew Reed, a certified health and personal development coach, entrepreneur, and author. My goal in life is to close the educational gap between science communication and the general public in order to make important knowledge and facts available to everyone. It is my mission to demystify the human brain by revealing how the body and mind influence each other, as well as how understanding these neurobiological processes can lead to a happier and more joyful life for anyone.

Over the past two decades, I have deeply immersed myself in research in the fields of neurobiology, psychology, health, nutrition, mindfulness practices, and personal development. Since then, I've helped innumerable clients unlock their maximum potential in terms of vitality, motivation, and health while giving them the tools they need to take matters into their own hands.

This is exactly what I will promise to you as, together, we embark on a journey to discover the most important pillars of restorative sleep and navigate around the numerous pitfalls and traps surrounding this fascinating subject.

I've pieced together this handy guidebook for anyone having difficulty falling asleep, staying asleep, and waking up the next day feeling fully refreshed and wide awake. My aim is to provide a practical scientific toolkit to upgrade your sleep hygiene, re-boost your focus, and enhance your overall drive and vitality. So even if you are not dealing with sleep problems directly, I guarantee that you will greatly benefit from improving your sleeping habits.

In this straightforward and practical guide, I will teach you how to hack your sleep for daily optimal performance. You will undo the abusive years—even decades—of self-neglect towards your health. I will explain how these various tools can ward off all the detrimental habits we've gained in our modern society. My aim is that the scientific toolkit in this book will aid anyone who:

- Suffers from restless nights of sleep or wants to improve their sleep-quality

- Has difficulty winding down and relaxing before bed

- Has lackluster energy throughout the day and frequently finds themselves irritable, frustrated, or groggy

- Cannot function without caffeine or a long-overdue 3-hour nap

- Has irregular sleeping hours due to work or other commitments

- Is interested in the science of sleep and its effects on their overall health and well-being.

Depending on your personal circumstances, you may have certain reservations. I can already hear some of my readers exclaiming, "But I've already tried everything; nothing has helped! Why should this time be any different?" – Please know that I am aware of your concerns. It's legitimate to feel disappointed if you've tried different approaches for optimizing your sleep without success in the past. This book, on the other hand, presents an in-depth and evidence-based solution to help you enhance your sleep hygiene. It does this by using the most recent scientific discoveries and providing practical guidance to support healthier sleeping habits. It also covers a broad range of ideas and strategies you've probably never even heard of before, while equally highlighting the importance of determining which options work best for you on an individual level.

Or perhaps it is the classic "I don't have time for..." scenario for those who are new parents, live with large families, or even those who work odd shifts throughout the week. While I understand that some people have extremely busy schedules, and some of the tools I'm about to present to you require a certain degree of planning, this book was written with the busy person in mind. It contains short, easy-to-digest chapters and actionable advice that can be implemented in as little as a few minutes per day.

Since it would probably take months for you to read all the research demonstrating the benefits of adequate rest to health and longevity, I've done the work for you and condensed it all into one handy guide. All I ask in return is that you allow yourself to reevaluate your priorities for a moment and give this much-neglected area the attention it deserves.

Because I guarantee, if you will start implementing even a single one of the following strategies, or better yet, layer a handful of them into your daily routine, you will notice a whole new sense of vitality, happiness, and well-being.

So, are you ready to discover the secrets to getting the best sleep of your life?

A Quick Side-Note:

The majority of these tools are easily accessible (there's no need to break the budget for your health) and readily available to you right now. While the intention is for anyone picking up this book to study it, layer each tool, and adopt a customized protocol to follow daily, it is, of course, up to you to decide which tips and advice serve your best interests. As far as I'm concerned, applying any one of these tools will undoubtedly hack your sleep and improve it indefinitely.

Sleeping: The Unappreciated Skill

The state of modern life is chaotic. We live in a thriving world designed to indulge our wants, but we forget that we've neglected our basic human needs. Despite the overabundance of resources at our fingertips, the lifestyle of the 21st century has some serious drawbacks:

Everything has become on-demand and readily available in the 21st century. We use apps every day for instant access to travel, fast food, and social connectivity. From streaming services that entertain us in the comfort of our own homes to online retail and grocery deliveries sent directly to our doorsteps,

We suffer from the paradox of choice every day as we decide what to consume from the thousands of options available to us. We pay more attention to how we appear and present ourselves to the online masses than to how we take care of our brains and bodies. We would rather work extra hours than have more time for ourselves and our families, dangerously upsetting the delicate balance between responsibility and leisure.

Along with this digital age enigma, other pressing health concerns have arisen all across the globe. Around the world, obesity rates have soared higher than ever before (Mitchell et al., 2011). Poor sleep quality is a widespread phenomenon that is still not taken seriously, even though it has been linked to a wide range of physical and mental health problems. Ultimately, these health crises are rising at an unprecedented scale, undeterred by the machinations of 21st-century living.

The convenience of consumerism may have been a drastic leap in human civilization that we're not equipped to handle yet. What was designed to make life easier for us has inevitably made it more burdensome. As a result, this fast-paced, on-demand world has thrown our priorities aside.

There is a wealth of evidence to support the multitude of reasons to sleep long and well. But without getting too ahead of myself, let me just say that sleeping is actually a difficult skill in the 21st century. There are so many factors that can potentially disrupt or impair the quality of our slumber, from the things we eat and drink to light intensity and temperature, to physical activity, all of which affect the effectiveness of our night's rest.

So it's not just our nighttime habits that we need to be cautious about.

Throughout the next couple of chapters, you'll learn to understand the fundamental nature of sleep. "Four Myths about Sleep" will examine the common misconceptions we all have surrounding the enigmatic essence of this state. "The Power of Slumber" highlights the numerous health benefits associated with a good night's sleep. "Gaining Control Over Your Sleep Rhythm" delves deeper into the mechanisms that run like clockwork every day of our lives to govern the sleep-wake state.

From there, the remaining chapters will provide the essential tools at different time periods and circumstances to help you get back on track with your sleep quality and duration. Finally, the book will examine some strategies that can be adapted to our 21st-century way of living, accommodating issues like jet lag, shift work, and even parenthood.

Naturally, it's difficult sometimes even for me to strike the right balance. We all occasionally succumb to our reliance on caffeine, naps, snacks, and other measures designed to keep us going when we can't seem to stay alert and focused during the waking hours of the day. As someone who struggled with his own health and sleeping habits for the first few decades of his life, I understand this challenge. Up until the age of 33, I wrestled with dopamine addiction, obesity, and low self-esteem. But in 2004, I decided to go on a determined journey of self-discovery, and in the end, I took responsibility for my own health. This is when I started reading up on the science of sleep, and eventually I came up with my ideal nighttime routine.

Now I'd like to reveal the toolkit that essentially saved my sleep and energy levels, so you can do the same. I'm a firm believer that we all deserve good, peaceful, deep sleep, and my wish for you is that you will greet each day feeling brand new and refreshed.

Quick Disclaimer

While I intended to write this guidebook with tools to hack any individual's sleep, I want to emphasize that this book will not help everyone. I am referring to those with chronic sleep disorders, such as sleep apnea, restless leg syndrome (RLS), and narcolepsy. If you have been diagnosed with any of these sleep disorders, conditions, or illnesses, please talk to a licensed doctor or a qualified health professional for personalized medical advice.

Additionally, the tools outlined in this guide focus exclusively on behavioral changes, including some nutrition and supplement advice. There won't be any mention of prescription drugs to aid sleep.

Dear Reader,

Before we begin, I'd like to express my gratitude for purchasing this book by offering my perspective on the never-ending pursuit of happiness as a small gift to you.

How to Ruin Your Life by Chasing Happiness

The 5 Surprising Habits We Think Lead to a Happy Life - But Actually Do the Opposite

Ain't we all chasing it, this elusive state that everybody is yapping about, yet no one seems to be able to pin it down - at least none of those who are trying so hard anyway. The truth is that happiness is a construct of our imagination. It's a feeling that we've collectively agreed upon as the holy grail of emotions. We've attached so much meaning to the word 'happiness', we've forgotten that it's just a word, devoid of any inherent value, much like 'flubbertidbids'.

By any chance interested in unraveling our self-sabotaging behaviors that lurk beneath the surface of everyday life? Well, my friend, you're in luck because my humble gift is precisely what you are looking for...

To get your free copy, follow the link below or scan the QR code on the next page.

https://matthew-reed.dualitybooks.com/free_gift

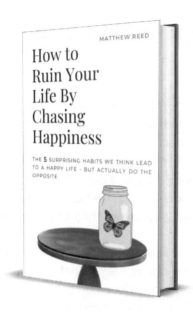

Simply Scan this QR Code With Your Smartphone's Camera and Download as an E-Book or Audiobook.

Enjoy!

Chapter 1: Four Myths About Sleep

So what do we know about sleep? Well, the science of sleep has been thoroughly investigated over the past couple of decades. We've learned about the significance of this state and the processes involved within the body during sleep stages. We've learned how sleep occurs and, more importantly, its far-reaching benefits for overall health and longevity.

However, at the same time, a lot of misinformation has been spreading online. Claims that imply that we need less sleep than ever before, can catch up on lost sleep, can be adapted to suit our needs in the modern age, and so forth. Although such claims have been disputed, it's important to reflect on the ideology behind them and learn to re-educate ourselves on what sleep really involves and why it matters for the general public.

As you might have guessed from the title of this chapter, I'm going to tackle the most common myths and debunk them once and for all.

Myth No. 1: Your Brain Rests While You Sleep

While it seems logical for the brain and body to rest during sleep, this couldn't be further from the truth. In reality, the brain is in an oscillating state during sleep. Instead of hitting the "power off" button and everything shutting down, imagine the brain entering a hibernation state. While our bodies get to rest and recuperate at night, our brain runs background processes and goes into housekeeping mode. Its job now is to keep the body's systems in good shape and make sure everything is running smoothly.

Now, this happens because the sleep phase occurs in five different stages. The first four stages are collectively called "slow-wave sleep." This is when our bodies enter the deepest, most serene state. The final stage is known as rapid eye movement (REM) sleep or "dream sleep." This is the most active sleep stage, and although most of our body is paralyzed by now, it is characterized by horizontal muscular twitches in the eyes that occur while we're dreaming (Patel et al., 2022). All this has been monitored in science by using measurements that specifically record electrical-brainwave activity in the brain, eyes, and muscles. Despite everything else being shut down, these areas of the brain still show activity when we enter the sleep phase.

Accordingly, when we go to bed and wind down for sleep, our brain prepares for this restorative phase. It works in intervals of roughly 90-minute cycles, working through the sleep stages described above.

During the first 30 minutes of the onset of sleep, we enter stages one and two. This is the introduction phase, where our bodies' internal systems are winding down. Here, things like heart rate get reduced and muscle tone relaxes. It's important to note that this is the lightest form of sleep in this phase.

In the next half hour, we enter stages three and four. This is known as the "deep sleep" phase, which is often associated with synchronized slow-wave sleep activity. Here in non-REM deep sleep, the brain mainly regulates the physical side of things: energy conservation occurs in the body, and the autonomic system maintains balance during this time, such as clearing up the toxic buildup of waste chemicals like free radicals from oxidative stress.

After 60 minutes or so have passed, we finally enter the REM sleep stage. This dream sleep allows us to regulate emotional processes and reflect on what has happened throughout the day; hence, learning and memory formation are primarily related to this stage (Siegel, 2005).

So, throughout the 90-minute sleep cycle, we have drifted from stage one to REM sleep. But it doesn't stop there. As the first cycle comes to a close, our brains and bodies oscillate back down from the REM sleep stage to stage one of slow-wave sleep, and this repeats throughout each successive sleep cycle. On average, we experience four to six sleep cycles a night

(Patel et al., 2022). In the first half of these cycles, we'll mainly experience deep sleep. Then, as we experience the second half of the cycles, we'll drift more into experiencing longer durations of REM sleep. Both periods of the night are critical since it's only the combined experience of deep sleep and REM sleep that ensures a restorative night's rest.

It's also important to note that I've simplified things by saying that the first four stages of non-REM sleep keep your body working and that the REM sleep stage helps you process your emotions. In reality, both stages maintain physical and mental function throughout our bodies. For example, growth hormone and testosterone production are maintained during the REM sleep stage.

There you have it! Our bodies may be resting in place, but our brains are maintaining law and order. By revealing the inner machinations of the sleep phase, I hope it highlights how important this one-third of our lives is for our longevity.

Myth No. 2: You Don't Need as Much Sleep as You Get Older

Based on what I explained above about brain activity and sleep cycles, it should be apparent why this myth is harmful. When we assume that we don't need as much sleep as we get older, we're sacrificing both sleep quality and quantity.

For instance, we think that children require more sleep for growth and development. But as soon as we reach adulthood, we're fully grown and developed by the time we're 25 years old; hence, this responsibility for sufficient sleep vanishes. But what many don't consider is that the sleep architecture of children differs greatly from that of adults.

As we grow older, the ratio of REM sleep drops gradually across our overall sleep architecture, while children experience a far greater amount of REM stage in their sleep during the same number of hours. However, this doesn't negate the importance of the REM stage for us as adults; in fact, it's still a vital stage in our sleep-wake cycles. We can't take it for granted. Therefore, it makes it even more significant to have REM sleep since it occurs infrequently in fragmented patterns throughout sleep.

Well, isn't that another burden of responsibility for adulthood then?

As I stated above, both non-REM ("deep sleep") and REM ("dream sleep") stages are crucial for restorative sleep. They both ensure good sleep quality and duration.

So if we were to sleep less often, we'd cause several of the following issues: we'd break one of several 90-minute sleep cycles, cause severe grogginess, disrupt either non-REM or REM sleep (depending on which half of the sleep phase we wake up from), and cause physical and mental dysfunction for the rest of the day.

In fact, the more we deprive ourselves of regular sleep, the more severe the effects of daytime drowsiness accumulate over time. While we think we'll adapt to this new lack of energy, this isn't the case. Depriving yourself of sleep on a regular basis can have serious consequences for your health, including an increased risk of cardiovascular disease, diabetes, impaired cognitive function, memory loss, weakened immune and fertility systems, and a host of other serious problems (Colten & Altevogt, 2006a).

But let's be honest here; I've done this too. I've not claimed to be a paragon of health who strictly follows these principles that I preach. I'm human, and I've adopted flawed behaviors in the past as well—these sleep myths exist for a reason. I think we always believe we're the exception to the rule. Throughout my 20s and 30s, I thought I could handle less sleep. In fact, I strangely felt proud of living off of a mere four to six hours a night.

But as I got older and reached my 40s, I found myself having to juggle the growing responsibilities of being a father and running my business. I still naively believed that at this stage in my life, I could handle a lot less sleep. After all, who needs sleep when I could spend more hours in the day being productive? Wrong. As the days and weeks flew by, I suddenly realized how ill-equipped I had become at balancing my roles at home and work.

Not only did this take its toll on my health, but it also impacted my relationship with my spouse. Another thing we don't realize is that by sacrificing that fraction of REM sleep in adulthood, our emotional processes suffer greatly. It didn't click for me that a lack of sleep quality could cause reduced empathy as well. This meant that a lot of conflicts in my relationship showed up more often, and both my partner and I would end up going to sleep in a frustrated state. Now, I don't need to point out how this hampered my sleep even further.

Overall, we need to ensure that we, as adults, sleep the recommended seven to nine hours a night (CDC, 2017). Following this guideline allows us to experience a range of four to six complete sleep cycles per night. Therefore, we gain the combined experience of deep sleep and REM sleep, which ensures a restorative night's rest.

Myth No. 3: You Can Catch Up on Sleep

This one actually felt all too relatable for me. For the longest time, we deluded ourselves by thinking that there was such a thing as sleep compensation. In other words, if we rack up a sleep debt over a day or so, we think we can undo the damage done by sleeping more on other days. It's that common thought we all share: "So what if I barely scraped by on three hours last night—I'll sleep an extra four hours tonight to make up for it." And so the story goes, again and again.

But we're actually doing more harm than good here.

Even if we manage to get some extra rest the following night and feel more alert and energized the next morning, this can cause havoc for the rest of the week. The circadian rhythm, our body's internal clock that regulates sleeping patterns, gets thrown completely out of sync. I'll explain more about this physiological mechanism in a later chapter, but, for now, I'll pinpoint why compensating for sleep debt is a bad idea.

In a nutshell, when we try to reverse sleep debt from last night, we're radically shifting our sleeping patterns. By compensating with additional sleep tonight, we end up doing one of the following: we go to bed earlier, wake up later, and leverage napping and caffeine intake to get there until that can happen.

By going to bed earlier, we've not accumulated enough sleepiness. Here's why: There's a chemical called "adenosine" in our bodies that gradually builds up during the day and causes the onset of sleep in the evening (Bjorness & Greene, 2009). This buildup essentially dictates when we should naturally fall asleep tonight. By going to bed earlier than usual, we're disrupting this threshold of accumulation. In other words, we won't feel sleepy if we go to bed at 8 p.m. instead of our regular time of 10 p.m.

Likewise, this happens when we wake up later the next day. Less of this chemical buildup will be present at the relevant times tomorrow. This means that it takes longer for it to accumulate and, therefore, it delays the onset of sleep. Basically, we won't experience our typical sleepiness until 12 a.m. instead of 8 p.m. See how this little adjustment in our sleeping pattern can disrupt our mood and energy levels over the course of more than one day?

Now, the tactics of napping and caffeine intake during this day of sleep debt will also cause disruptions. If we consider what I discussed above, napping also disturbs this chemical build-up that we need to make our circadian timing work properly. Even these short bouts of rest will agitate sleep tonight. Also, caffeine blocks this buildup and delays sleepiness in other ways, so this solution is not good either. However, that isn't to say that both these tactics are useless—they're just ineptly used the following day after a really bad night's sleep. In later chapters of this book, I'll talk about how napping and drinking coffee can be used to great effect.

For now, we just need to realize that we can't compensate for sleep debt. As of today, the only solution is to do nothing. In this best-case scenario, by doing nothing differently the next day, we can safely induce sleepiness, fall asleep quicker, and stay asleep longer tonight. While this is shocking to hear, it's one of those situations where we have to knuckle down and battle through the temptations. Otherwise, we compromise our sleeping patterns in the long term.

Myth No. 4: Sleep Timing Doesn't Matter

This one may be difficult to read about for night-shift workers and new parents, but, unfortunately, when we sleep is just as vital for our health. Homeostasis exists in us human beings for a reason. Our sleeping patterns are rigid and can't be muddled up; otherwise, they can disturb the delicate internal balance in our brains and bodies.

To highlight this point, I'll touch lightly on our circadian rhythm again (that internal clock that you'll be hearing a lot about throughout the "Sleep" section). Although I'll explain the underlying behavior of this physiological mechanism separately in its own dedicated chapter. This internal clock governs our bodily systems over roughly a 24-hour cycle. Several elements that we experience in our immediate environment have an impact on this.

During the day, our levels of alertness can vary depending on things like the amount of daylight and the temperature. However, interestingly enough, our circadian rhythm has evolved to self-govern us, even in the absence of such environmental factors.

There have been several case studies involving individuals isolated in darkness for long periods of time (Mills et al., 1974; University of Chicago Library, 2016). From what they observed in cave experiments, our circadian rhythm still runs its course independently and governs our activity state over the same 24-hour cycle (Mills et al., 1974). Even in remote darkness, it still tells us when to be awake during daylight hours and when to fall asleep during night hours. Fascinating, isn't it? In these experiments, however, the subjects' circadian rhythms were thrown off for about an hour longer than usual (University of Chicago Library, 2016). But even with this additional time, this internal clock deprived of light managed to adapt accordingly and still retain its homeostatic mechanism.

So, if in darkness our internal clocks can still dictate when we're asleep and awake, how does this affect our modern lifestyle? Well, it means that if we're up in the middle of the night for whatever prolonged reason, we're agitating the delicate order of our bodies. Likewise, we upset the balance if we're asleep for most of the day. Studies have shown that working night shifts disrupts sleeping patterns and can lead to reduced immune system functioning and cognitive abilities (Kazemi et al., 2016; Liu et al., 2021). Furthermore, these individuals are prone to developing what is known as "shift work sleep disorder" (SWSD), which can make the workers more susceptible to judgment errors, impaired mental functioning, and other health issues (Wickwire et al., 2017).

Now, I know this is alarming news. However, I'm also aware that the vast majority of us can't abandon our responsibilities and neglect our livelihood. We can't afford the luxury of quitting shift work or dropping our parental obligations. While it's vital to sleep according to our natural rhythms, not everyone can maintain a semblance of balance between being alert during the day and asleep at night. But all is not lost. I've shared some hopeful strategies in the last chapter of this book for those stuck in these circumstances.

All things considered, we've observed the tip of the iceberg. By examining these misconceptions surrounding sleep, it's apparent that this state is severely misunderstood. While we know it's crucial for great health, how does snoozing benefit us? What does sleep specifically do for our brains and bodies? Let's dive deep beneath the surface to find out how far the iceberg lies.

Chapter 2: The Power of Slumber

It's fascinating to uncover what happens when we sleep, isn't it? In the previous chapter, I outlined the important neurobiological processes behind this state. But now I want to discuss the wide-reaching implications sleep has on our general health.

Let me explain exactly what sleep does in our day-to-day lives.

Sleep and Longevity

This may feel like a no-brainer at this point, but better sleep significantly improves our lifespan. What we don't realize about the sleep state is that various systems in the body are running discrete operations. Internal feedback loop mechanisms are in place to ensure homeostasis in all aspects of the body so that we can rest and feel refreshed the next day.

But these neurobiological operations can only happen through a network of gene expressions that oversee everything. Imagine that our genes are supervisors regulating quality control on the factory floor. So if we experience sleep deprivation, the correct genes can't be activated and perform their duties properly. If there's no leadership to oversee the smooth background operations, then it can become catastrophic quickly.

Gene expression must be maintained to coordinate cellular rejuvenation and other vital processes such as immunity, metabolism, cell division, neural development, and hormone levels. Studies have discovered that our DNA—the genetic material of life—gets damaged on a daily basis (Lindahl & Barnes, 2000; Branzei & Foiani, 2008). So sleep is essential to repair the damage that has accumulated over the course of the day.

Furthermore, sleep prevents cellular aging. Remember chromosomes—those pairs of cross-shaped bundles of DNA strands that contain the genetics we inherited from our parents? Well, they're susceptible to damage as well. At the ends of our chromosomes, there exist molecular regions of DNA sequences called "telomeres" (Zhu et al., 2018). They are essentially the "protective caps," much like aglets on the ends of our shoelaces. Not only do they protect our precious chromosomes from being frayed, but they also serve as the staging ground for cell division. However, every time telomeres divide, they get shorter.

Accordingly, as the telomeres on the chromosome ends shorten, they accelerate cellular aging. This is because cell division is a vital process in the human body, and without it, many aspects of our health can be compromised. Fortunately, they get replenished by a special enzyme that prevents such disastrous consequences. Yet, this can only happen if we get sufficient quality sleep on a regular basis.

Sleep as a Reset

Sleep is well-known to act like a deep reset for the day. It's a state designed to rejuvenate our health in so many aspects. However, this has far-reaching effects on our happiness, drive, emotional stability, concentration, and mental sharpness. In fact, it has been shown that better sleep quality drastically enhances psychological well-being (Hamilton et al., 2006). So there's no denying the interconnectedness that sleep has on a whole host of physical, mental, and emotional health conditions.

For example, it is known that growth hormone (GH) stimulates development in several areas of the human body. It supports the growth of bones and cartilage in childhood and plays a role in healthy brain function by influencing hormones like insulin and affecting blood sugar levels. While I could write an extensive list about this hormone's benefits, I'll leave it there for now. More importantly, it has been revealed that there is something called a "sleep-onset GH pulse," which induces the release of this hormone as we enter slow-wave sleep (Van Cauter & Plat, 1996). This happens during sleep as GH aids in tissue repair and metabolism changes that occurred during the day.

Similarly, testosterone is also secreted while we sleep. It plays a crucial role in both men and women, serving to increase libido, repair muscle mass, fat distribution, and bone density, as well as improve brain and heart health. This hormone also rises when we first fall asleep, and its levels only start to peak during the first bout of REM sleep in the night.

In fact, both testosterone and GH are responsible for the muscle-building properties we acquire from a good night's rest. When we sleep well, both these hormone levels rise and begin the process of tissue repair and regeneration, which, therefore, helps us recover post-workout. Not only would we lose the ability to build muscle if we didn't get enough sleep, but the resulting hormonal imbalance would also cause depression, fatigue, and other problems.

Sleep, Memory, and Cognitive Function

Imagine the following scenario: It's a new work week, you're in the office, and you sit for endless hours as you work on a project deadline that is due this Friday. Throughout the day, you're grinding away, typing and sipping, sipping and typing, taking bathroom breaks, heading out for lunch, typing once again... until eventually you clock out at 5 p.m. and retire for the evening.

Except you forget to save and back up all of your work.

When you return the following Tuesday morning, you discover that none of your work is there. It doesn't exist! All your due diligence is thrown out the window. You sit down and grind again, furiously praying that it won't happen again. You clock out at 5 p.m. and retire for the evening... until Wednesday morning comes and you discover the exact same thing happened. You inquire about it with your colleagues, but they shrug and don't notice anything wrong with their work—it's all backed up to cloud storage.

One even chides, "Have you tried turning your computer off and on again?"

You try again on Wednesday, only this time you have less gas in your tank. The work ethic shrivels up, and little to nothing gets done.

This keeps repeating day in and day out until, eventually, Friday morning arrives. Now you're stuck in a room with your superiors as they wait impatiently for your presentation to begin the meeting. However, there is nothing to show for your hard-earned efforts.

This is what happens to our brains when we deprive them of sleep. You see, the brain relies on solidifying everything we've learned in a day when we rest for the night. From our general day-to-day experiences to skill acquisition and all other relevant knowledge gained in a single day, our memory systems are a database of information. However, they require time and energy to be able to transfer the relevant stuff from the short-term freight trucks to the long-term warehouses for processing.

So, when we suffer from sleep deprivation, we're dismantling the highway for these trucks to travel across safely.

For memory formation to occur, neurons (i.e., type of information messenger) have to strengthen their communication with one another. They typically do this at the gap junctions between their nodes, known as "synapses." Here, the trucks (or "vesicles") have to unload their cargo of neurotransmitters (chemical communication between nerves) into this bay and send them across to the next neuron. However, for synaptic plasticity to occur, the neurobiological signal must exceed the activity threshold (Kandel et al., 2012).

The function of sleep allows this activity to ignite across synaptic receptors; hence, these vesicles can dump their contents across them frequently. Whee synaptic communication is strengthened enough over a period of time, it reinforces the long-lasting effect of signal transmission between neurons. When this development happens, it is called "long-term potentiation" (LTP), a process that is linked with learning and memory formation (Kandel et al., 2012).

So, where does cognitive function fit into all of this?

Well, we've discussed how memory is where you save and back up your brain. But the cognitive function is the part that greases the mental gears, allowing you to work and do your due diligence for the day. When we deny these mental faculties by sleeping less than the recommended amount, we experience cognitive decline (Alhola & Polo-Kantola, 2007). We're unable to think clearly or remember events properly, and we're vulnerable to neurodegenerative diseases like Alzheimer's. For instance, it has been shown that the cumulative effects of cognitive decline make us susceptible to developing the biological hallmarks found in this notorious disease that gradually develop into brain plaque (Peter-Derex et al., 2015). So it's worth winding down properly to back up the important information from your day.

Sleep and Immune Function

Speaking of memory, did you know that sleep plays an intuitive role in the formation of immunological memory? Yep, much like how GH is released from the initial onset of slow-wave sleep, it also contributes to accelerated immunity. Specific immune cell levels rise higher in the bloodstream, which is particularly beneficial in creating a defensive response when we're sick.

Sleep and immunity seem to coexist in a mutually beneficial relationship. One affects the other, and vice versa. As the sleep stages unfold, our bodies free up more activity so the immune response can get to work. Our immunity is split into two categories: innate and adaptive. The innate side regulates the periodic inflammation that we develop in our bodies, sending out the relevant cytokines (i.e., immune cells) to carry out various tasks. The adaptive side, meanwhile, pulls together its resources and searches the whole bloodstream for any foreign threats that need to be taken care of (Janeway et al., 2001). The immune system responds in a coordinated way to make sure we stay safe and healthy.

Accordingly, when we're sick, our immune responses crank into high gear. Our sleep actually alters itself to accommodate the immune system's defenses against infection. We purposefully enter stages of sleep that use the least energy, so our immune system can turn up the fever and promote the march of its infantry cell units to deny the pathogen's advances. Interestingly, this response often happens during REM sleep, and the fragmented experience of this stage for the immune defense system is what causes fever dreams.

Now, if we were to deprive ourselves of sleep, it could drastically affect our immunity as well. For instance, it has been shown that less than six hours of sleep can reduce the number of natural killer cells (another type of immunity-based cell) by 75% (De Lorenzo et al., 2015). Furthermore, the disruption of a normal sleeping pattern can also have detrimental effects. That is why the World Health Organization (WHO) recently classified night-shift work as a possible carcinogen due to its negative impact on our immunity (IARC, 2020).

Sleep and Mood

There's a sound reason for our sudden crankiness after a sleep-deprived night. Numerous studies have demonstrated that people who are sleep deprived report having worse moods (Triantafillou et al., 2019).

Not only that, but sleep issues are also associated with several types of mental illnesses, including depression and anxiety (Goldstein et al., 2013; Nutt et al., 2022). For these conditions, similar to immunity, it tends to be cyclical, where sleep deprivation or excessive sleep is a cause as well as an underlying symptom.

This is because when we don't get enough REM sleep, our ability to deal with emotions and remember things is greatly reduced. Because of this, it's difficult to remind yourself of the good feelings and memories you have on a given day. Additionally, as we experience mental illness symptoms, a negative feedback loop is set off, which results in more insomnia and, ultimately, a downward spiral of detrimental effects on our general health and wellbeing.

While this lack of sleep causes difficulties in emotional processing and behaviors, it also affects our judgment. Sleep deprivation can increase the incidence of accidents in the workplace or mentally engaging activities like driving (Kazemi et al., 2016). The increased drowsiness affects our abilities to make rash decisions and lowers our mood, so we're unable to think clearly and make good decisions. So it's not just the way insomnia affects us, but how it affects those around us in our environment as well.

It goes without saying that chronic insomnia worsens mental and emotional disorders and can push people toward suicide. Therefore, it's crucial that we understand all of these wider health implications that sleep has on various aspects of our health.

How Much Sleep Is Enough?

Hopefully, by now, it's clear how vital sleep is for various aspects of our health and well-being. As was said above, it is the key to living a long life because it controls many things that help our memory, brain function, immunity, mood, and mental health.

But how much sleep is enough for us to get the benefits of the deep reset it provides?

Experts agree that adults should aim for an average of seven to nine hours of sleep a night. While children (depending on their age) should get nine to fourteen hours of sleep (CDC, 2017), I can't stress how equally important sleep quality is alongside sleep quantity. Even if you get the recommended seven hours of sleep a night, you may be falling into one or several pitfalls and traps that are disrupting your sleep architecture.

Quality is also the key to success here.

This ensures that we enter all the appropriate stages of sleep. We want to move into the deeper non-REM and REM stages so we can get all the health benefits listed in this chapter. After all, if we can rejuvenate overnight, then we're guaranteed to feel refreshed when we finally wake up.

Throughout the rest of the book, I'll be highlighting tools and strategies that will both improve sleep quality and duration. If we want to experience the multitude of health benefits mentioned above that sleep grants us every night, then please pay close attention to the following chapters.

Chapter 3: Mastering Your Sleep Cycle

By now, you're familiar with everything sleep provides us for our health and well-being. You may have also noticed that I keep referring to things like sleep rhythm and timing. But what exactly does this mean?

Sleep rhythm is the pattern that governs when we're awake and when we're asleep during a typical day. More importantly, there's a way for us to leverage the tools within this book so we can control the timing of our sleep rhythm. But first, I want to explain the sleep-wake cycle further so we know intuitively which neural and hormonal systems we're influencing with these strategies and tools. Throughout this chapter, you'll learn who the key neurobiological players behind our sleep rhythm are and the underlying mechanisms they control.

If we consider a tree's roots to be neurons (i.e., nerve cells), we can understand how our nervous system works. The roots in any tree anchor it into the ground to keep it firm and stable. By the same token, they also act as the senses beneath the surface: the roots absorb any nutrients in the soil and amplify the growth and development of the tree itself. Therefore, this integral channel system acts as the foundation for the tree's life support. Similarly, we couldn't function without our nervous system since it's hardwired throughout our brain and body. Overall, the nervous system acts as the mediator for the entire process of the sleep-wake state.

This is important to bear in mind as we delve into the rest of this chapter. Now let's plunge into a deep dive into neuroscience!

The Circadian Rythm: Your Inner Time-Keeper

In a nutshell, two forces—circadian and chemical—determine our sleep-wake cycle. Both of these forces directly influence the neurobiological mechanism inside all of us known as "the central clock." This clock is a brain region called the "suprachiasmatic nucleus" (or SCN) and is located in the hypothalamus—the homeostatic control center in our brain that ensures the lawful nature of sleep (Ma & Morrison, 2022).

First, let us explore the meaning behind the „circadian force".

The term "circadian rhythm" actually describes biological cycles that the body has been genetically programmed to repeat every 24 hours (Andreani et al., 2015). This time-dependent physiology governs our behavior through environmental cues, which determine when we're awake and when we're asleep. Therefore, this is the driving force responsible for governing our internal sleep-wake state over the course of a day.

However, peripheral clocks in organs and tissues as well as a network of "clock genes" tightly control this complex system on a feedback loop (Sukumaran et al., 2010). The expression of such genes determines important internal events circulating in our bodies: things like our metabolic activity, hormonal levels, and other processes in the nervous system. Since this circadian force is coupled with a genetic network of levers and cranks to stabilize everything, it reinforces its influence on the network as well.

Our circadian rhythm alters the majority of our gene expression. This has a whole host of implications for our health since gene modulation is integral to controlling everything that happens in our bodies. For this reason alone, it's essential that we master the natural laws of our sleep rhythm.

As you will soon discover with all these underlying mechanisms, the circadian force primarily responds to sunlight. Light is the MVP in our sleep-wake state. It sends signals to our bodies that wake up our senses and move the gears in the central circadian clock. While sunlight is the main influence that grounds our sleep-wake state to normal rhythms, there are other key factors that also play a crucial role.

Whenever the SCN is ticking away and coordinating the body's responses, another structure is feeding other inputs into this circadian clock. This is the intergeniculate leaflet, and it monitors several signals affecting the body, such as temperature, exercise, meal timing, and even drug intake (Moore & Card,

1994). Hence, this clock gets fed different sources of information from both our environment and our internal states (more on this later).

Overall, there is a powerful pacemaker effect that keeps all of the body's circadian functions and mechanisms stable. It's neat how there are barriers regulating every stage of the sleep-wake process—kind of like the red tape of bureaucracy in a way.

Next, I'll explain how these mechanisms underlying circadian forces work in tandem with a chemical force to set the central clock's timing over the course of a typical day.

Cortisol: Hack Your Inner Alarm Clock

As dawn rises and the sun ascends overhead, the light poking through the curtains hits our eyelids. More specifically, light enters the retinal ganglion cells in our eyes and hits the melanopsin photoreceptors (Hattar, 2002). This environmental cue communicates important information from our eye sockets to our brain, telling us that it's time to wake up. Our inner alarm clock is about to be primed. As you might have guessed, our circadian central clock is what causes this response.

Now, the relay race of information commences. The SCN begins its daytime duty and informs the body to wake us up via the control center, the hypothalamus.

This part of the brain sends this message from the brainstem to all the relevant connected systemic pathways in the autonomic nervous system (Jones, 2019). This involves alerting all the organs and tissues in our body to begin preparing for the waking state.

We then receive the waking signal from both the hormonal and neural responses in our body. One of our organs, the adrenal gland, produces a small amount of the hormones cortisol and adrenaline. Now, these hormones are associated with the perils of stress, particularly the fight-or-flight survival response during dangerous situations. Adrenaline raises heart rate and blood pressure, while cortisol boosts energy resources by increasing glucose availability and uptake in the bloodstream. This may not seem like a useful expenditure of resources, but it's a surprisingly effective strategy.

Here is why a little bit of stress in the morning is actually a good thing: The key lies in the fact that only a small amount of cortisol and adrenaline are released from the adrenal gland. This quick waking signal response is colloquially called the "cortisol pulse" (Benz et al., 2019). These low levels are enough to break us out of sleep's spell and arouse us into alertness without causing any harm. By stimulating all the usual suspects (organs and tissues) involved in fight-or-flight situations, our body is kicked into high gear to begin a new day. Also, the fact that this all happens in such a short time frame is truly remarkable.

So now our inner alarm clock has provoked us into an

alert and awakened state in the morning. But the story doesn't end there. The cortisol pulse may be the first key player in the central circadian clock's scheme. This is the first responder to make us readily available in the mornings. But what happens as the day goes by? Who then takes charge? More importantly, who's involved in drifting us back to sleep tonight?

Adenosine: The Body's Natural Sleep Aid

The moment our cortisol pulse awakens us, another process begins. In the background, a "sleep timer" has been activated within the hypothalamus. In twelve to fourteen hours, a combination of chemical mediators will induce drowsiness and make us fall asleep tonight. These homeostatic forces involved in this marathon toward sleep are adenosine and melatonin. The former is the driving chemical force and is signaled by the internal cues of our bodies' biochemical processes, while the latter is a messenger from the circadian force that helps us wind down.

Both forces work together to set the neurobiological stage for sleep.

Meanwhile, the SCN is ticking the seconds away until that happens. After all, it has to ensure that everything happens on time and according to schedule.

Now let's first examine adenosine, the chemical force that drives our hunger for sleep in the evenings. As we go through the day, we accumulate sleep pressure from this chemical enforcer.

I'll briefly explain why: When we wake up from the circadian force, our body has a lot of stored chemical energy called adenosine triphosphate (ATP) (Bonora et al., 2012). This is the energy currency that we generate through nutrient consumption, and we use it for essentially everything. This energy fuels healthy functioning and development throughout our lifetime. As ATP gets used for everyday life activities, it breaks down into a product known as adenosine. As the hours go by, adenosine levels gradually build up, and when the evening comes around, we feel incredibly sleepy.

This buildup of adenosine activates sleepiness throughout our bodies by means of a "lock and key" mechanism (Bjorness & Greene, 2009). To put it simply, the "keys" of the adenosine chemicals fit into the "locks" of their corresponding receptors. As a result, the push-pull lever mechanisms for the sleep-wake response get triggered. In other words, some types of adenosine receptors trigger brain areas that power down and reduce levels of wakefulness, and vice versa for other types of adenosine receptors that elevate levels of sleepiness.

Finally, as the adenosine levels accumulate, the sleep pressure rises higher and higher. By late evening, our hunger for sleep is ravenous. It gets to the point where it's harder to stay awake at night (although we may resist in vain). While adenosine is responsible for the relentless onslaught that diminishes our energy levels, it isn't working alone to achieve this victory.

The Yin and Yang Hormones of Sleep-Balance

As an army of adenosine besieges our fortress of alertness, melatonin employs discrete methods of infiltration. It sneaks behind the walls to open the gates for the ravenous horde of sleep mongers.

Melatonin is a hormone that bides its time over a 12- to 14-hour interval while we're awake. During daylight hours, serotonin production is stimulated. This is a beneficial neurotransmitter that is produced through either direct sunlight or the breakdown of the amino acid tryptophan, which is commonly found in our diet (Pandi-Perumal et al., 2005). Serotonin regulates our overall mood and temperament, but it is also one of many neurotransmitters that play a vital role in maintaining our focus and attention during the day.

While you may be asking why we're discussing serotonin right now, trust me, there's a reason for it. You see, light inhibits melatonin. This means that during the day, a light signal suppresses any form of melatonin production. Conversely, it is in the darkness where melatonin thrives.

As soon as dusk arrives and the sun sets low on the horizon, melatonin makes it move. In the darkness, an organ called the pineal gland produces enzymes that dismantle serotonin. By stabbing the neurotransmitter in the back, they break down serotonin, and melatonin is produced from the conversion. Under this guise, the darkness hormone ignites the torch for the sleepy signal. It's important to note that melatonin can only operate under dark conditions. Since the hormone is extremely sensitive to light, its presence will inhibit it.

Melatonin, in general, promotes the body's natural transition into sleep by increasing adenosine production. This has the cumulative effect of suppressing wakefulness and tipping the scales in favor of sleep. It also gently nudges our circadian rhythm to align with the natural cues of darkness, hence reminding us that we need to rest tonight.

Now the late evening has arrived. The combined circadian and chemical forces of melatonin and adenosine are victorious. Both of these sleep signals travel through our bloodstream and turn on the right neurobiological switches to make us less alert and more drowsy. But this could only happen with the appropriate cues: the external dark environment and the internal onset of general fatigue.

Ultimately, our sleep-wake state should be naturally aligned with the rhythms of the day. Both external and internal cues govern our energy levels and inform our bodies about the best course of action.

How Stress Can Disrupt Your Sleep-Wake Balance

In a nutshell, the SCN's concerted effort coordinates every homeostatic mechanism in the autonomic nervous system. This central clock determines the chronological order of events for our natural sleep-wake state. Every aspect of these neurobiological affairs needs to happen accordingly. Yet, in our modern society, we've managed to upset this delicate balance. I want to discuss here the potential implications that arise when we mess with the natural order of all this.

So we know that our brains have a central circadian clock that is the master switch for controlling the sleep-wake state. From the information it receives from the circadian and chemical forces mentioned above, it communicates signals across the bridge between the hypothalamus and the brain stem. From there, the signals are sent downstream to peripheral clocks in our organs and tissues, as well as to the clock gene network. So it's a tightly woven system that creates a cascading effect throughout the body.

Let's take a look at an example of how this system can be disrupted. Stress is one concern that tampers with the circadian system. Before we dive into it, it's vital to know that in the circadian rhythm mechanism, the hormones cortisol and melatonin have a connection. Since cortisol keeps us awake by sending signals to the peripheral clocks through the autonomic nervous system, it is the messenger that keeps us awake. In the same way, melatonin keeps us sleepy through similar pathways, including the autonomic nervous system. It's the messenger that tells our bodies' clocks to wind down. Naturally, this means that cortisol levels drop when melatonin levels rise and vice versa. One hormonal pathway gives up the reins for the other to succeed in its place. This is how the cortisol-melatonin dynamic relationship coordinates effectively at the appropriate times.

However, when we suffer from chronic stress, this throws a wrench into the delicate balance. Stress that becomes chronic can cause inflammation, raise blood sugar levels, weaken the immune system, and cause other problems that have a big effect on our circadian rhythm. Cortisol levels remain unnaturally high, and this imbalanced response means that there are no typical dips and peaks at the right times of the day. Therefore, cortisol's usual response becomes blunted, making it difficult to perform its duties properly. This inevitably affects the opposing rhythms of melatonin, and the hormone is thrown into abnormally high levels of production as well.

Ultimately, the cortisol pulse gets suppressed, and we don't get the appropriate signaling for waking up in the morning. Likewise, the unwinding effects of melatonin are blunted in the evenings, so we can't fall asleep at the appropriate times. Overall, we get out of sync with our bodies' natural circadian rhythm, which is bad for our health. This is why stress can have disastrous results in the long term.

There are also situations where the chemical forces

are altered. While we'll later discuss the antagonistic relationship between caffeine and adenosine, there are other health issues that affect this mechanism. For instance, underlying diseases and health conditions can promote excess production of adenosine, which could involve suppression of the immune system, tumor growth, pain, and inflammation, as well as being a hallmark indicator of brain and psychiatric disorders (Borea et al., 2017).

In conclusion, we've discussed how chemical and circadian forces influence the sleep-wake state. Throughout the day, these mediators interact with mechanisms all throughout the brain and body. By first educating you with this knowledge, you will recognize how all the following tools and strategies in this guidebook are designed to leverage these neurobiological processes to your advantage. I have no doubt that the rest of this book will optimize your performance during the day and improve your sleep quality significantly.

With this in mind, let's dive into the first tool in this book.

Tool 1: The Days Before Matter

Whether we are aware of it or not, how we feel when we wake up is a result of our actions over the previous few days. If we want to succeed at forming new habits with the toolkit, we have to examine our current habits first. It's vital to look at our past daytime and nighttime behaviors. By doing this beforehand, we can figure out what we individually do on a daily basis that hampers our chances of success.

In a journal, I want you to record your behaviors over the course of a week. Be honest with yourself–there's no judgment here. It's important to analyze what you do on a given day. After all, these habits accumulate over the week. Write down detailed answers to the following list of questions below:

- How do you feel this morning?

- How many hours did you manage to sleep?

- What did you do this morning when you woke up?

- Have you been outside today?

- What kind of meals did you eat? How did they affect your energy levels?

- How much caffeine and alcohol did you consume today?

- Did you manage to fit in some exercise? If so, what time did you exercise?

- What activities did you do in the evening?

- How did you wind down for the night?

- How do you feel tonight?

- Did you wake up at any point in the middle of the night?

Aim to record a daily log for about a week. From there, and as you read through this guidebook, you will be able to pinpoint any behaviors that are hurting your sleep. There are many habits that we've developed in the 21st Century that affect our sleeping patterns. Therefore, it's ideal to recognize such disruptive behaviors early on.

Additionally, there are effective sleep trackers available to us in the modern digital age. Wearable devices such as the Oura ring, Whoop 4.0, and the Biostrap are designed to record our biometrics. Similarly, there are also apps like Rise, Sleepscore, Sleep ++, and Sleep Cycle that are all especially useful in precisely tracking our sleep behavior. We can utilize these digital tools to monitor our current sleep quality and duration. This ensures that we can address glaring issues in our sleeping patterns over the long term.

Conclusion

Because our behaviors are such an individualized experience for each of us, this tracking tool can identify exactly which critical period of the day we need to focus on. The combination of using a journal and digital trackers to record our habits and behaviors will make it much easier to see what we need to fix. By pinpointing where we are currently at with our routines, we can address the problems with our sleep deprivation quickly.

Chapter 4: Perfect Your Morning

Let's now address the rest of the sleep toolkit in these chapters. Many of these hacks are designed to play to the strengths of our circadian rhythm. By using them, we can send the right neurobiological signals throughout the day and optimize our sleep accordingly.

Here I'll start laying the groundwork for a perfect day. There are three important timing frames in a 24-hour period that we can use to our advantage:

1. The morning to midday period (e.g. 6 a.m. to 12 p.m.)

2. The afternoon to evening period (e.g. 12 p.m. to 6 p.m.)

3. The late evening to night period (e.g. 6 p.m. to 12 a.m.)

Of course, this schedule fluctuates depending on your work occupation and geographical location. Focus on what you can do during these critical periods of the day, from the moment you wake up to the moment you wind down for sleep. This ensures success in making your sleeping pattern restorative again.

This chapter will now delve into the first critical period of the day.

Make Sunlight Your Best Friend

From what we've discussed about the circadian rhythm in the previous chapter, light plays a critical role in our biological evolution. The sun is the primary "time giver" that dictates our internal 24-hour clock.

To briefly explain, I'll use a simple analogy for nutrition: Every cell in our body requires energy for survival. We supply this in the form of nutrients we ingest, like organic food molecules. These chemicals get broken down into component parts in our gastrointestinal tract and are delivered to the cells via the bloodstream.

Similarly, the cells in our body also require light. This gets supplied to us in the form of photons we absorb from sunlight. When we detect this information, it sends an electrical signal through our retina. The melanopsin cells (aka photoreceptors) on the inner retina transmit this signal to variously specified neurons. Eventually, this gets delivered to our body's cells via several pathways in the autonomic branch of the nervous system.

It is through this optical input mechanism that we're able to bridge communication between all systems involved in the circadian rhythm. From there, the SCN will either wake up or shut down the neurobiological areas that control sleep and wakefulness, depending on what time of day it is.

The neurons in these neural pathways are very sensitive, and they respond best to the light spectrum that occurs at sunrise and sunset. Overall, the light intensity throughout the day determines whether we're alert or drowsy at certain times. Therefore, it's vital that we realize how beneficial sunlight is for us.

Tool 2: Ditch The Snooze Alarm

Though it may be tempting to hit the snooze button on your alarm clock, it's not worth the hassle. This is because our sleep cycle gets interrupted the minute our alarm goes off. As we've discussed, from the moment our eyes open, our body has already begun priming itself for alertness. So hitting snooze and returning to sleep for a few minutes won't help us—our sleep will be fragmented and won't feel restorative at all. That's why we inevitably enter a groggy state, even though we may have hit "snooze" several times already. The architecture of our sleep has been dismantled, and the body knows intuitively (from physiological cues) that it's time to commence the day.

Additionally, we're just hyperactivating the stress response in our bodies. The brain sends yet another cortisol pulse into our system because it anticipates that the next snooze interval will wake us up suddenly again. This repeated action will inevitably activate the fight-or-flight response in the morning, which will only make things worse. So, trust me, the snooze button is not worth it!

Instead, it's better to set your alarm for the latest

possible time that you have to get up. This ensures that you get more restorative sleep and avoid making that groggy state worse first thing in the day. If you can't resist the urge to hit snooze, then definitely place the clock further away from your reach. When the alarm goes off across the room, this forces you to get up, walk over to it, and turn it off.

In the process, you're more likely to be awake by this point. This is the critical moment when you should head to the bathroom and commence your typical wake-up ritual. To increase your odds, set your morning alarm to a melodic tune. It's been shown to reduce our perception of grogginess when we wake up (McFarlane et al., 2020). Meanwhile, the groggy state that we all experience will eventually wear off after half an hour. This is far better than experiencing excessive grogginess for the rest of the day.

Tool 3: Watch the Sunrise

So, we're finally awake and out of bed. With all this attention on circadian rhythm and light intensity, you might have guessed that it all begins in the morning.

During the first two hours after waking up, we need to go outside and see direct sunlight. I cannot overstate how critical this tool is for our alertness. The ideal time for early sunlight exposure is around sunrise, since our melanopsin cells are especially sensitive to the light spectrum then.

Now, obviously, it's difficult to be awake at the crack of dawn. So instead, it's better to focus on the next best thing: all we have to do for this tool is simply be outside and view natural light whenever the sun is up overhead. Yet, I must highlight that it's important to be outdoors in the fresh air and not just view the morning rays through a window. According to some studies, the photoreceptor stimulation and UV radiation in our eyes are significantly reduced if we only view sunlight through glass (Almutawa et al., 2013).

Nonetheless, it's important to keep in mind the duration of this practice too. Depending on where you live, the season, and the density of cloud cover, this affects how long you should spend outdoors in the morning. These factors all influence the available light conditions, so I'll give rough estimates on this for each situation.

If it's very bright outside, five minutes should be plenty. On a typical cloudy day, 10 minutes should suffice. However, if it's extremely cloudy and dismal, we need to spend roughly 30 minutes outside to get the benefits of this tool.

While viewing the morning sunlight, I want to emphasize caution: please don't stare directly into bright light! This can hurt and even damage the retinas in your eyes, so I advise against it. You shouldn't experience any discomfort while viewing light, and you should never look directly into the sun. Instead, aim to get peripheral light in around you—that should be plenty to get the intended benefits.

By just being in the vicinity of sunlight first thing in the morning, we drastically improve our alertness. The tool helps in two ways: 1) the morning light turns on your photoreceptors, and 2) the fresh air gives your body oxygen. I have no doubt you'll already feel more awake and alert for the rest of the day.

Tool 4: Time Your Exercise

Now, I don't want to harp on much about the health benefits provided by regular exercise.

We all know that exercise is fundamental for longevity. The heart's ability to pump blood with oxygen and glucose is important to our brain's ability to function. By being physically active, we increase our heart and lung health. Intense aerobic exercise is good for the cardiovascular system because it improves blood flow and makes the heart and arteries stronger. Ultimately, this leads to improved blood flow and, hence, increased nutrient uptake by the brain. In a nutshell, a strong heart and lungs equal a healthy brain.

There's a reason that we've been prescribed 150–180 minutes of moderate aerobic activity per week (WHO, 2022). Naturally, these effects play into our sleep conditions as well. Studies have shown that regular exercise promotes overall sleep quality (Dolezal et al., 2017). This is due to the aftermath effects of exercise invoking earlier melatonin release, which thus contributes to the shift in circadian rhythm timing. This expedites the onset of sleep—we get sleepier much quicker in the late evening and are fast asleep before we even know it.

It doesn't matter what kind of exercise activity we do daily. Whether you prefer aerobic, resistance, mobility, and flexibility, a bit of balance work, or a combination of each type, it will all provide a significant boost to your overall health.

For myself, I combine my love of the great outdoors with some physical activity. This already layers two of the tools in the morning: viewing the sunlight while you exercise can give tremendous, reinvigorating results. For instance, during the week I settle for short morning walks among nature. In Vancouver, you can almost always find me strolling through Stanley Park. But almost every weekend, I embark on hiking adventures throughout the nearby regional parks. The mountains and valleys are so beautiful that I can't help but want to go exploring. I even convinced my family long ago to join me on these weekend retreats, and they have now become a staple tradition in our household. Generally speaking, it's wise to find a physical activity that nourishes you so it can become a sustainable habit in your daily routine.

However, the timing of exercise is also important here.

For most people, age and underlying health conditions play a critical role in exercise timing. Typically, it's ideal in these situations to exercise in the mornings and early afternoons so our bodies wind down quicker in the second half of the day. This will keep us energized and alert as we go through the rest of the day's trials and tribulations. It also ensures drowsiness at the right times later in the evening.

Although evidence suggests that exercise in the evening doesn't negatively affect sleep quality, this is only the case in certain situations (Alley et al., 2015).

We must avoid performing high-intensity exercise close to bedtime; otherwise, our sleep will be harmed. Furthermore, we should avoid being active in the final couple of hours leading up to bedtime. This is because, after exercise, we get a rush of endorphins and our core body temperature rises. It takes many hours for these to drop back down, and as a result, we feel more alert than tired in the evenings. So, as long as we don't break these two cardinal rules, our sleep won't suffer tonight.

Conclusion

In essence, this is how the first critical period of the day should flow. Using these simple blueprints, we can feel more refreshed every time we wake up. The timing of these tools in the morning will optimize our performance throughout the rest of the day.

Chapter 5: Maintain a Productive Day

Meanwhile, we're transitioning into the second critical period: the afternoon shift leading into the early hours of the evening. Here, we want to stay the course to maximize our energy and peak performance.

However, at this point, it's crucial to remark on the concept of "circadian dead zones," which are basically buffer zones in the day where our circadian rhythms can't be shifted by things with light exposure—to an extent. They often coincide with the rising phase of our core body temperature, which naturally aligns with the time period when we're most alert. Typically, someone experiences these moments during the first half of this second critical period.

Although this may be true, the following tools should be used with caution. If we don't consider the timing and moderation of these tools, they can be improperly used and have a dire effect on our sleep. Since it may not seem like they initially alter our sleep-wake state, in reality, the delayed consequences reveal themselves when we try to wind down at night but can't seem to ward off our active nature.

As long as we abide by this, then the following tools can be leveraged to great effect.

Tool 5: Employ the Tactics of Napping

Who knew that the Spaniards had it right this entire time? While many of us may scoff at the idea of napping during the day, it's not just a Spanish cultural tradition. There are actually proven benefits to taking a siesta in the afternoon.

When they're done right, naps can provide tremendous perks for our health (Mantua & Spencer, 2017). Also, in even as little as ten minutes, we can experience several cognitive benefits from napping.

There's no point in resisting the fact that we all experience that afternoon dip. It's that moment when we get that slump in energy and the bed looks more enticing than ever.

But you can battle it out all you like; sooner or later, you'll crash. Our energy levels aren't infinite. We've already seen how adenosine accumulation oversees this. That's where the saving grace of napping comes into play. A nap during the afternoon can range from anywhere between 20 and 90 minutes. The timing depends on the type of benefits you'd like to gain from this short bout of rest.

However, before you hop into bed or lie like a log on the couch, there are some caveats to point out. Firstly, this is where it's important to highlight individuals' differences. For some people, napping works wonders for them. But for others—particularly those who suffer from insomnia—I generally wouldn't recommend it, as it can make sleeping at night far worse. So, only keep reading if you are a person who gets a good night's sleep and occasionally enjoys a nap.

Secondly, we need to be aware that napping affects the buildup of adenosine in the brain. This means that the typical sleepiness that should be induced by the evening can get delayed or lost since the adenosine buildup gradually depletes during napping. While this sounds like incredible news, it means that sleep onset can get delayed too. In other words, we may risk experiencing insomnia if we time our naps incorrectly.

Thirdly, if we nap for a significant amount of time, it can cause "sleep inertia" (Hilditch et al., 2017). This is that short window of grogginess we experience when waking up from rest. So if we time it longer than what is recommended and interrupt a sleep cycle, we may cause up to an hour or so of grogginess afterward. That certainly won't benefit anyone if we're trying to optimize performance throughout the day.

Thankfully, we can avoid these worst-case scenarios.

If we want to prevent insomnia tonight, don't nap too late in the afternoon. The latest you want to time your naps is roughly six to seven hours before bedtime. For instance, if you're planning to sleep at 10 p.m., have your nap at the latest between 3 and 4 p.m. Next, to avoid grogginess, make sure you limit your nap to about 20 to 25 minutes. Even though longer naps are better for you as an individual, if you sleep for more than this short amount of time, you will probably feel groggy.

In addition to this, we can couple our napping routine with a dose of caffeine for good measure. By getting some caffeine before a nap, we can help get rid of sleep inertia when it's time to get up. Now who wouldn't want an extra boost in performance from this deadly combo?

Regardless of how you choose to tailor your napping schedule, what matters here is that we deploy this tool into our routine. A worthwhile short rest in the afternoon is a small price to pay for optimizing peak performance.

Tool 6: Avoid Sleep-Saboteurs

Unfortunately, there are several ways our nutrition affects our sleeping habits. By eating less of the following foods, we can improve the structure of our sleep cycles in a big way.

Even so, I'm not suggesting that anyone needs to eliminate these dietary choices from their lives forever. Rather, it's important to understand why these have a profound power over sleep. We can also learn how to limit the impact that these things have on our energy and performance.

Caffeine

As you may have already guessed, caffeine is one of the notorious substances that abuse our sleep– especially when we drink it after 2 p.m.

Caffeine is a devious assailant. When we drink our coffee, tea, or other caffeinated beverage, the molecules of caffeine block the adenosine molecules' receptors. Basically, this means that the correct key (adenosine) can't fit into its lock and, therefore, it can't send the signal for sleepiness at the appropriate times.

You may be thinking as you read this, "This is brilliant news; I can just keep sipping on caffeine and never feel tired again!" However, this is misleading.

There's a reason for the well-known "caffeine crash" we all experience. Although caffeine nudges adenosine out of the way and guards the gates to slumber, it is only a temporary effort. The adenosine levels still build up quietly in the background. When caffeine levels slowly dwindle over many hours, the adenosine receptors start becoming accessible again. By this stage, adenosine has accumulated a lot. So after eight to ten hours, when our caffeine levels have dropped to a quarter of what they were, these receptors will be flooded with adenosine, which will make us feel very tired. This is when we're overwhelmed by tiredness and we're compelled to go to sleep right away.

Despite this consequence, I know you think there's an easy strategy here: you'll be tempted to consume caffeine and time the moment to hit the hay when that big dip in energy happens. But you're forgetting that caffeine still exists in tiny levels in your body. When we finally drift off to sleep, the leftover caffeine in our system disrupts the stages of non-REM deep sleep. Ultimately, our sleep quality is compromised, and we inevitably wake up groggy the next day. Then our reliance on caffeine for energy increases, and this vicious cycle of dependency gradually increases.

None of us wants to get to the stage of drinking six to eight caffeinated beverages daily. Especially when the maximum recommended intake is around 400 mg a day (Harvard School of Public Health, 2020). Since it lingers in our system for a while, it's better for you and your sleep cycle if you don't consume caffeine after 2 p.m. as a strict rule. This will give the caffeine enough time to leave your system when you wind down for your bedtime routine. So the list of caffeinated substances includes the common culprits like coffee, tea, sodas, and energy drinks. But it's crucial to know that caffeine is also found in chocolate, energy bars, guarana, and painkiller medications. So consume these sparingly during the day.

Alcohol

As much as we all love to have a drink every now and then, alcohol does have negative effects on our sleeping habits. The substance sedates us into a drowsy state by enhancing adenosine production and can help us fall asleep quicker. However, the major concern here is what happens after the alcohol effects wear off.

When alcohol levels drop in the middle of the night, it leads to fragmented sleep. This means that we inevitably wake up frequently throughout the night (whether we're aware of it or not). These repeated awakenings shorten our quality of sleep; hence, we always feel awful after drinking the night before.

Additionally, alcohol greatly disrupts our REM sleep. This has severe implications since REM sleep is linked to learning and memory formation, as well as general emotional processing for mental health (Purves et al., 2001; Colrain et al., 2014). There has even been a link to a decrease in growth hormone release during REM sleep (Prinz et al., 1980). If alcohol is repeatedly abused every night, it could make someone's mental health significantly deteriorate, and it may even increase the risk of developing psychiatric disorders (Colrain et al., 2014).

Nonetheless, this isn't to say that we have to stop having fun in our lives. We all can still have our evening plans to socialize and enjoy occasional drinking. Having a pint at lunch or a glass (or two) with dinner won't kill us. But remember that it can take roughly an hour for our bodies to metabolize just one serving of alcohol (Cederbaum, 2012). So the advice here is to try and limit alcohol consumption in the remaining few hours before bedtime. By doing so, we can manage to mitigate the negative effects on our sleep—not to mention the nasty hangover the next morning.

Diet and Meal-Timing

Did you know that everything you consume in a given day can impact your sleep quality? Well, that's unfortunately the case: nutrition not only has an effect on mood and cognition, but it also impacts our sleep and energy levels throughout each day.

Studies have shown that a low-fiber, high-saturated fat diet reduces the amount of deep, restorative sleep (St-Onge, Roberts, et al., 2016). Furthermore, any excess sugar we have can also increase the frequency with which we wake up in the middle of the night (St-Onge, Mikic, et al., 2016). This is because these types of foods in our diet also influence blood glucose spikes. Overall, that means there's a drastic reduction in sleep quality if we eat a lot of processed food in our diets.

Also, if we eat a heavy meal very close to bedtime, our digestive system will take a toll on our sleep as well. This is because the digestion rate slows down when we enter sleep, so any excess food or food that is difficult to digest quickly can upset our stomachs when we lie down. It can lead to issues such as indigestion and acid reflux that make falling asleep even trickier. If possible, avoid eating heavy meals close to bedtime. Things like greasy takeaways or high-fat, high-protein foods like red meat are best eaten earlier in the day. The latest time you want to eat your last meal is three hours before your usual bedtime.

But don't let this news discourage you. If you get hunger pangs late in the evening, you can still eat a light snack. For example, seek out a nutritious snack that contains B-vitamins and L-tryptophan, which helps induce the production of melatonin.

Cannabis and CBD

I just wanted to briefly mention other recreational substances here. While cannabis and CBD may be legal in certain parts of the world, they can also have a negative effect on sleep.

While there have been proven short-term benefits to aiding sleep in those with insomnia, cannabis also affects sleep quality (Kuhathasan et al., 2019). The THC component in cannabis (aka the psychoactive component) can impair REM sleep similar to alcohol. So the regular use of this drug can have a bad influence. Furthermore, if the individual stops taking it as a sleep aid, there may be severe repercussions from experiencing rebound insomnia.

Contrary to this, CBD may not have as much of a negative effect on sleeping. However, it has been shown that CBD promotes wakefulness even at low doses (Wiginton, 2021). These are just some facts to bear in mind; I advise that anyone using these substances should do so at their own risk.

Tool 7: Watch the Sunset

As I previously mentioned, our circadian rhythm is hardwired to a 24-hour cycle. In the presence or absence of light, our internal clock resets and dictates when we should naturally be awake or asleep at a given time of the day.

It makes sense then that the ideal timing for us to re-experience natural light is around sunset. This is because those melanopsin cells that I mentioned in the "Perfect Your Morning" chapter are extremely sensitive to changes in light intensity. These cells transmit light activity received by the photoreceptors and communicate to the internal SCN clock what time of day it is.

Hence, that's why it is so important to go outside around sunset, preferably for a short walk, so your body adapts to the evening hours of the day. If possible, you can aim for another round outside, this one lasting a half hour.

While you may be skeptical at first, there is some reasoning behind the madness: the sun is an integral cog in the sleep-wake cycle. In the morning, sunlight is bright overhead and emits a blue wavelength of light that stimulates and revitalizes us (Wahl et al., 2019). While in the evening, sunlight hangs low on the horizon, and the sunset emits red wavelengths of light that relax us and promote the production of melatonin (Wahl et al., 2019).

This in turn will help induce sleepiness into our system as our circadian rhythm resets for the day. So do yourself a favor and step outside one last time today— your sleep will thank you for it later.

Conclusion

When used together, these resources provide dependable power through the day's toughest hours. It's during this second critical period when we all hit the afternoon slump and self-medicate to persevere with productivity. Yet, we can re-learn how to keep our energy stable in smart ways by just breaking bad eating habits and getting over the shame of taking a nap. Finally, we shouldn't forget the importance of sunlight when the transition to evening commences. Our internal clocks need the signal to set the appropriate wind-down time tonight.

Just a Quick Question on the Side...

Do you find value in what you're reading or listening to and would you consider leaving an honest review of this book? It won't cost you a thing, just a quick 30 seconds to share your thoughts with others. Your voice can go a long way in helping someone else find the same inspiration and knowledge that you have.

If you're not sure how to leave a review for an Audible, Kindle, or e-book, it's easy! For Audible, just hit the three dots in the top right of your device, click rate & review, and leave a few sentences about the book along with your star rating. For Kindle or e-readers, just scroll to the last page of the book and swipe up to find the review prompt. And if you're reading a physical copy of this book, simply head over to Amazon and leave your review there. If you scan the QR code below, it will take you directly to the review page. It's that simple!

Thanks so much for considering my request. Your feedback means the world to me, and it will help others discover the same joy and inspiration that you've found in this book.

Chapter 6: Fall Asleep Like a Pro

Okay, we've reached the final critical period. In this chapter, I'm going to show you how to practice good sleep hygiene for the remainder of the day. The following nighttime tools will address all the pitfalls and traps that we've all succumbed to either in the past or currently face in the present.

At this point, the morning has passed and you have followed the protocol mentioned in the previous chapter. As the daylight shifts into the twilight hours and the evening gathers, your body will be naturally primed to do the same. But in this modern age, we've fallen prey to a 21st-century lifestyle that overstimulates our senses.

Whether you believe it or not, you'll soon learn and realize just how damaging our current habits are to our sleeping patterns. The tools laid out here will shed insight into the harmful behaviors we've adopted. Through natural means, we can strive to achieve some balance and make our sleep restorative again.

Tool 8: Simmer Down

So at this point you must have realized that the brain doesn't have an "off switch". The brain still runs in hibernation mode at a lower power capacity. It's vital, then, to consider the brain as having a dimmer mode in the darker hours of the evening.

But the problem with this mode is that it makes it easy for the brain to get too much stimulation from the environment. This becomes a problem, especially after dusk.

In the evenings, the photoreceptors in our eyes have a high degree of sensitivity to light intensity. In other words, they require very little light to stimulate us and keep us alert and awake. While this contradicts the high sunlight exposure we need in the mornings to stimulate our body, the opposite is true later in the day. Unfortunately for us, this means that we must avoid artificially bright lights as much as possible.

Sounds impossible, right?

Thankfully, it doesn't have to be complicated. Studies show that we just need to avoid any color and intensity of bright artificial light between the hours of 10 p.m. and 4 a.m. (Tosini et al., 2016). So we don't have to sacrifice our evening leisure completely, just for a few short hours when you would normally be asleep anyway.

All we have to do is signal to our brain that it's time to wind down for the night. This would involve habits like dimming the lights in your home when possible. For example, it's more preferable to use low-level lighting like lamps instead of ceiling fixtures. You can even use candlelight on tables or depend on moonlight (although that could be tricky if you're planning to cook).

Furthermore, it's recommended to spend the three hours before your bedtime doing relaxing activities instead of energizing ones. It's best not to engage in stimulating activities since they keep our senses awake rather than allowing us to wind down properly. To clarify, we should avoid the following habits late at night: things like playing video games, watching action, thriller, or horror movies and TV shows, doing an intense workout, and even arguing with our partner or family before heading off to bed.

Look, I know it's not ideal to hear this. But it's a small compromise to make to improve our sleep quality, which is what we are aiming for here, right?

Before you begin watching that next episode of your favorite binge-worthy show, maybe turn off the TV and unwind from all electronic devices. Or another option could be to adapt the light intensity settings on your devices in the evening hours. There's a reason why we've become transfixed to our screens. They've been designed to optimize our attention—so screens are not an ideal companion for our bedtime routines.

Every screen on every device we use emits a blue light. This specific type of light has the effect of keeping us focused and alert, but it also blocks melatonin production. Yes, that's right—all these devices actually prevent us from feeling sleepy and heading off to bed at appropriate times. That's why it's also crucial to adopt the method of using blue-light filters in the evenings. This can range from setting up free software like Flux, which adapts your monitor's screen light to natural lighting conditions during the day, to setting light filter options on your phone, tablet, and TV as well. If you can afford the luxury, there are also blue-light-filter sunglasses that are specifically designed to aid with this effect during the evening hours. There's also the option of dimming screens or even setting some to "grayscale" mode, but I imagine that's for those hardcore folks out there who don't mind viewing a lackluster screen in black and white for the rest of the night.

Tool 9: Craft a Bedtime Routine

Be proud of yourself that you've avoided the "sleep-saboteurs" so far. It is perhaps the most difficult tool to apply, along with "simmering down" in the evening with relaxing activities. These are no easy feats to achieve since our current living environments aren't designed for enhancing our sleep at all.

Here comes the next difficult step: adopting a consistent bedtime routine that you can follow every night. Naturally, as human beings, it is significant for our circadian rhythm to set a consistent sleep and wake-up schedule every day. Not only will this tool anchor your 90-minute sleep cycles and prevent sleep quality from being interfered with, but it will also aid you in getting the recommended sleep quantity every night.

For example, if an individual went to bed at 10:30 p.m. every night and woke up at 7:30 a.m. every morning, they'd acquire the ideal upper limit of nine hours of sleep. By doing this same thing every day for a few months, you can build a strong base for your sleeping pattern.

Of course, this is easier said than done.

Even after applying the previous tools in the toolkit so far, we may still struggle to fall asleep quickly. But a bedtime routine makes this less of a problem by sending the right neurobiological signals to our systems and getting us ready for sleep. Sooner or later, we need to safely land into slumber.

So how do we develop this evening ritual?

Well, first we need to set a realistic time for when we want to sleep. For instance, consider what other factors are involved: Do we have other family members or partners to be mindful of? When do we start work the next day? How do we like to spend the first few hours of our morning for ourselves?

As we think about these circumstances, it'll help us set realistic expectations. However, we must avoid taking extreme measures with our sleep regimen (unless there's a non-negotiable obligation behind your reasoning). Going to sleep at 8 p.m. and waking up at 4 a.m. is not a realistic expectation. Then again, neither is going to sleep at 2 a.m. and waking up at 10 a.m.

When we've chosen a time to go to bed, the wake-up time should always be in line with the recommended "seven to nine hours" of sleep (CDC, 2017). Please keep this all in mind when figuring out the appropriate schedule for yourself. Now that we've designated a consistent sleep and wake-up schedule that we can stick to long-term, let's focus on the finer details.

Next, let's turn our attention to what we do in the final hour or two before we actually head to our bedrooms. The beautiful thing about this is that the bedtime routine should be tailored to our lifestyle. While certain aspects should be regimented, like the bedroom environment, other aspects of the bedtime routine can be modulated.

The method I like to envision is one that focuses on three fundamental components: taking care of your bedroom, taking care of tomorrow's nagging concerns, and taking care of yourself.

Let's look at this through the lens of a hypothetical scenario below.

I've decided that I want to go to sleep at 10 p.m. every night. First, I set a reminder in my calendar: the hour before bed is when my bedtime routine begins. By the time nine p.m. arrives, I've taken the appropriate sleep supplements (see "Tool 14" later in the book), and I'm ready to begin my evening ritual.

First, we take care of the bedroom. My wife and I

ensure that our room will be dark, quiet, and cool. We draw the drapes and make sure there isn't a peep of light poking through. There is immutable silence, aside from the city's background noise outside the windows. Finally, the room is well ventilated. At this point, it's very important that we turn off and unplug all of our electronic devices. We both turn off anything that might wake us up in the middle of the night with a notification.

Secondly, I take care of any nagging concerns for the next day. I pick out my outfit and set it up somewhere close by, prepare some of my breakfast and work lunch, and even add water to the stove-top kettle to save some time in the morning.

Finally, I practice unwinding with therapeutic activities. For myself, this either involves a quick yoga stretching routine, meditating for a few minutes, or perhaps even journaling my thoughts and concerns onto paper. Afterward, I sip on a cup of chamomile tea and read some of the sci-fi novels that I have left idle on my nightstand—the curiosity of what happens in the next chapter is enticing. Eventually, I floss and brush my teeth with my wife, say goodnight to our kids, and turn off any remaining dim lighting before we tuck ourselves into bed and fall asleep.

This happens around the same time every night. By following a set pattern of behaviors, we're sending encouraging signals to our body that it's time to wind down for sleep.

For these reasons, it's crucial that you personalize your bedtime routine to suit your needs. Arrange your bedroom so it's accommodating for a good night's rest. Take a few moments to quickly prepare a few things for tomorrow. But above all else, make time for self-care and do activities that nourish your well-being. You have to craft a pre-sleep routine that is both sustainable and pleasurable, so you can consistently follow it every night before your appointed bedtime.

Tool 10: Keep It Cool

For a successful night of sleep, there's one aspect we need to ensure: the temperature of our bodies. Now, I know at this point you're thinking, "Matt, I've already done all the above steps, and you're telling me that my good night's sleep is still not guaranteed?" On the contrary, I point out this tool because it may disrupt your sleep during the night.

Rest assured that this tool is equally important. By regulating our body's core temperature, we can fall asleep quicker and avoid being disrupted in the middle of the night. In the hours leading up to sleep, our core body temperature already drops gradually. This is because temperature is a biological signal for the circadian rhythm, which makes melatonin and makes it easier to fall asleep every night (Harding et al., 2019).

For effectiveness, we need our bodies to drop their core temperature by 1-3 °F every evening.

This occurs through glabrous skin portals on our body—the face, ears, palms of our hands, and soles of our feet—which allow for increased blood flow and regulate heat. It is in these body areas that we can allow for "vasodilation," or the body's cooling mechanism, to reduce our core body temperature later in the evening (Wong & Hollowed, 2016). These extremities allow for quick heat loss, making it easier to cool down and induce the transition to sleep quicker.

Perhaps it's best to not skip this step after all?

The core body temperature is around 98.6°F (37°C), but this fluctuates by a couple of degrees in the middle of the night. To ensure that our bodies cool off for a good night's sleep, we must make the bedroom temperature range between 60 and 65°F. The last thing you want is for your bedroom to be too hot, as those sweltering conditions will cause sweating and reduce deep slow-wave restorative sleep significantly (Okamoto-Mizuno & Mizuno, 2012).

One method is to have a hot shower or bath before bedtime. Yep, you read that correctly. It's because this increase in temperature actually thermoregulates our core body temperature as a result. When we step out of the tub, our bodies begin this natural cooling effect via the glabrous skin areas. This is one perfect way to aid sleep. We can help this cause even more by setting the thermostat, using a fan or air conditioning, keeping the curtains closed at night, opening the windows for air flow, or even using seasonal bedding to fit your needs. Basically, do whatever you can to cool your body down and fall asleep.

You'll know if you're not cool enough when you stick a limb out of the bed covers in the middle of the night... and, well, just hope you don't have that scene from Paranormal Activity embedded into your head. Otherwise, you'll find yourself quickly retracting that limb and suffering the rest of the night with nightmares.

Conclusion

All things considered, the tools disclosed in the final critical period form an integral part of a typical evening. When combined together in a night routine, they can be wielded to great effect. While it may seem like we're sacrificing our leisure time, we need to reframe these techniques as gentle reminders for winding down. Indeed, they can be staggered at different intervals across the night to provide the right behavioral cues for our body's clock.

Chapter 7:

Tools for Dealing With Sleep Interruption

Just like in life, even if we've done everything right, things may still go wrong. It could be the case that we've fallen asleep right on schedule and woken up in the middle of the night. Or it could be the case where we're tucked into bed but can't seem to drift off.

Ironically, I'm writing this chapter after my own sleep has been interrupted. So don't worry; you're not alone in dealing with this.

Generally speaking, it's very common to have frequent sleep interruptions as we get older. Adults are predicted to wake up at intervals summing up to 30 minutes or more (Mander et al., 2017). So, unfortunately, it comes with the territory of aging. However, this frequent waking is fragmented throughout our sleep cycles during the night. We shouldn't be experiencing longer periods of wakefulness during this period.

That is why in this chapter I want to tackle those issues that creep up and affect our ability to fall asleep in the first place or wake us up needlessly longer than anticipated. At the same time, while we attempt to use these tools, it's important to avoid blue light in the middle of the night to prevent overstimulation of the senses. That's the last thing we need when trying to fall back to sleep.

The "Bathroom-Break" Type

This is yet another issue that comes with the territory of aging. Admittedly, I never thought I'd fall into this category. I'd always scoffed at the idea of my grandparents getting up several times in the middle of the night to relieve themselves with a toilet break.

But fast-forward a couple of decades later, and I'm right where I didn't want to be. Again, I want to reiterate that as we age, it's perfectly normal to frequently wake up—especially if it involves a quick trip to the bathroom. It is a condition known as "nocturia," which simply refers to frequently waking up because of the urge to urinate (F. Duffy et al., 2015). The important thing is that we bounce right back into our usual sleep cycle after a short amount of time being awake.

Although, there might be an easy fix below if we find ourselves going to the bathroom far too often at night.

Tool 11: Sip Your Last Beverage Instead of Gushing It Down

One quick behavioral change involves the way we

drink. Many of us don't realize that drinking a lot of liquid in the few hours before bedtime can upset our bladder. This is because ingesting a lot of any beverage in a short time frame can trigger the bladder's neural response.

In other words, the excess liquid sloshing around in your system stimulates the kidneys and bladder to get rid of it immediately. In that case, it's better to not only curb drinking any beverages close to bedtime but rather to lean toward sipping them slowly instead of gulping them down.

Similarly, it's also crucial to avoid any liquids that are categorized as "bladder irritants." These are the usual suspects that I mentioned in Chapter 5 when discussing which drinks to avoid earlier in the day, like caffeine and alcohol, but they also include other diuretics like citrus fruit juices.

Ultimately, these tactics slow down stimulation of the bladder's neural response and may, in fact, save you that extra trip to the bathroom tonight.

The "Active-Mind" Type

Come on, admit it—you've attempted to just lie there, on your back, staring at the ceiling, but your defiant body tosses and turns anyway. Meanwhile, your brain is hyperactive and plans out the meals for tomorrow as well as every single errand and task that needs to be done. Oh, and by the way, it never fails to conjure up another thought or two. This is a common scenario, especially in modern times.

While at this point many of us turned to desperately counting sheep, the mental arithmetic makes things far worse. Since we're engaging a part of our brain with stimulating activity, this makes it even more difficult to fall asleep. Instead, it's more practical to learn how to calm our minds. That being said, settling and calming our minds is not an ability we are born with but rather a skill that we must hone.

Tool 12: The Ritual of Mindfulness Practice

Mindfulness is a skill that is often neglected. Over the decades, I spent a lot of time refining this aspect in my own life. I've found it to be tremendously invaluable in my lifestyle today. There are various health benefits highlighted in mindful practices, such as yoga and meditation. Findings have shown physiological changes in the autonomic nervous system that promote a more relaxed response in the body (Nagendra et al., 2012). The reason for this being that mindful activities lend themselves to reduced stress, heart rate, and blood pressure while also helping to regulate serotonin and melatonin release for sleep.

While you are suffering from nighttime anxiety, I encourage you to do one of the following exercises: guided meditation, Nidra, using a breathing technique, or visualization.

I want to focus on guided meditation, which has become more and more popular in the digital tools space. There are several apps these days like Headspace, Balance, and Insight Timer that provide an intuitive, user-friendly experience for all newcomers. I'd highly recommend checking out any of these guided meditation apps since they serve to make the transition to mindfulness practice much easier. All you have to do is listen to the audio recordings, and they'll lead you through the breathing exercises in a step-by-step manner.

Similarly, Yoga Nidra is a form of yogic sleep that follows the principles of guided meditation. It soothes and transitions us to a calm state by focusing on affirmations, visualizations, and systemic relaxation in every limb of the body. Specifically, this type of practice focuses on drifting us through the four states of brain wave activity that happen during the sleep-phase cycle. If you're having trouble relaxing before bedtime, try one of the many free guided yoga nidra sessions available on YouTube.

Finally, if you're already familiar with mindfulness practices, you should try visualization. This would entail certain techniques that involve walking in a comfortable environment. Ideally, pick somewhere safe and secure that grants you tranquility. Spend some time imagining yourself in this place, much like the guided mindfulness practices we talked about above.

Each of these techniques involves lying face-up in bed anyway, so you're already halfway there! However, if you're uncomfortable with the idea of breathwork, I'd encourage you to start with guided meditation sessions as they're easier to handle. Remember that there is no right or wrong way to practice mindfulness. It's essential to know this as we delve into these kinds of activities for their therapeutic benefits.

The "Insomniac" Type

I think we've all been there. Everyone has experienced insomnia to some degree in their life. For whatever reason it may be, we simply can't fall asleep no matter what we do. Contrary to the notion that we must buckle down and try falling asleep harder, we actually need to do the exact opposite.

It could be useful to have a cathartic outburst with a proverbial pen and paper. While we may have already journaled during our bedtime routine, inherent thoughts still creep up on us at night. The problem with ruminating on thoughts is that their magnitude increases tenfold during the night. Consequently, as Dr. Matthew Walker aptly put it in a podcast interview, "We need to shut down the emotional tabs in our browser" (Huberman, 2021b). So, it's better to pick up the journal again and write down every nagging worry and concern circulating in our heads. By simply compartmentalizing these thoughts somewhere else, it gives our headspace some room to breathe.

To add to this point, it's not worth lying awake in bed for half an hour. Although we all pray for the soothing embrace of sleep, we can't force it—even with the help of all these tips and tricks. It's far better to leave the vicinity of the bedroom and do a relaxing activity. This could be the journaling mentioned above, but it could also involve reading a book or doing breathwork—anything that can help calm and ground the mind again.

In due time, we'll find ourselves wandering back toward the bed. It might be worth revisiting the previous tools mentioned in "Fall Asleep Like a Pro." Is your environment still quiet, dark, and cold? Try to find a way to address these issues. In the case of abrupt noise from elsewhere, we can try using earplugs to help soothe us into sleep. Although some people report them to be uncomfortable, so it's a matter of trial and error (Karimi et al., 2021). If there is ambient light poking through, we can wear eye masks to shield our vision. However, it's worth mentioning that the mask shouldn't be too tight, as that can affect breathability in the lustrous skin on your face. With attention to temperature, we must keep the room and ourselves well-ventilated: open the window or turn on air conditioning, and maybe elevate your feet to change the circulation in your body and help it cool off.

Finally, one crucial bit of advice that I once got from a close friend was to remove all clock faces from my bedroom. While our phones should be neatly tucked away in silent mode, far away from us, we often forget about the alarm clock. Its LED glare showcases that perpetual reminder that it's already very late, and that classic concern rears its head: "If I fall asleep now, I'll only get 'X' amount of sleep.'" When we know the time in the middle of the night, it exacerbates our stress further. We all have important events cropping up every day, but we don't need that nagging reminder of time ticking away in the background. So please aim to turn its face away from your line of sight; it'll do wonders for your health.

Conclusion

Generally speaking, we want to plug the leaks causing our sleep interruptions as they happen. By remembering how the mechanisms of sleep and circadian rhythm work, we can leverage this new insight to our advantage. In effect, they'll support us in our endeavor to fall back to sleep and stay in this remarkable state for the rest of the night.

Chapter 8:

Adaptive Strategies to Boost Your Success

Now, in a perfect world, we'd follow all these guidelines flawlessly. But the fast-paced demands of our environment make it difficult, if not cumbersome, to use the practical tools and strategies in an ideal setting. Our modern world is notorious for neglecting good sleep practices in favor of efficiency. So it's no surprise that you may be skeptical about what you can use from this guidebook and adapt it into your own life.

That being said, it's not impossible to adapt this sleep toolkit and leverage it to our advantage in different scenarios. There are physiological cues from both our body and the environment that we can manipulate in our favor. To do this, we need to consider biological concepts like chronotypes and the underlying factors that govern sleep and wakefulness mentioned throughout the book so far.

By paying close attention to these important factors that affect how we sleep and wake up, we can deal with social and travel jet lag, night shift work, and even the sleepless dangers of being a parent. Finally, we can then bolster our chances of success further with the aid of sleep supplement stacks as well.

Let's dive in. By collectively using the tools we've learned so far, we can adapt to any climate.

Chronotypes

So you may have heard of the terms "night owls" and "early birds," perhaps even "hummingbirds" as well. These are all categories of a biological concept known as a "chronotype." These concepts are behavioral expressions underlying our circadian rhythm that determines our varying levels of sleepiness or wakefulness during the day (Raman & Coogan, 2019). In fact, evidence suggests there's a strong genetic component involved in chronotypes that affects some of our clock genes that regulate the circadian rhythm (Lane et al., 2016).

For one thing, it accounts for the individual differences we experience with one another. Depending on our age and gender, chronotypes can widely influence our routines. They dictate why teens inevitably sleep in as they go through the woes of puberty or why the elderly always wake up and fall asleep at insanely early hours.

Chronotypes remain the fundamental difference between each and every one of us. Some of us always feel groggy waking up at 7 a.m., even after a full night's sleep. On the other hand, some people may always feel wide awake in the late evening hours when those around them are ready to snooze.

No matter how much we resist them, these differences are naturally hardwired into our internal clocks. Ultimately, chronotype also greatly influences aspects such as our appetite, activity levels, and core body temperature throughout the 24 hours of the day.

While we can train our circadian rhythms with the toolkit, our chronotypes are more rigid. Also, chronotypes aren't simply split into three categories; they exist on a spectrum. Some studies have identified chronotypes under labeled categories like "bear," "wolf," "lion," and "dolphin" to account for individual differences among populations (Lindberg, 2020). But more importantly, we can determine our own chronotypes through self-assessment. There are a plethora of online questionnaires that can help you shed light on your typical behavioral patterns.

It's essential to figure out which chronotype you have, since this will help you leverage this guide's toolkit to maximum effect. Our chronotypes determine things like the time period of our peak performance, our eating habits, and when we should wake up and fall asleep according to our natural rhythms. With this knowledge, we can optimize our performance during the day. With the help of your chronotype and this toolkit, you can change these aspects of your circadian rhythm and make them fit your schedule. This will undoubtedly prove useful in the scenarios below, where we'll adapt strategies based on everything we've learned so far to improve our health and quality of life.

Tool 13: Use Your Core Body Temperature as an Anchor Point

Even if you don't notice it, your body temperature changes slowly throughout the day. This is because of the sleep-wake cycle. For example, when we're experiencing sleepiness, our core body temperature is at its lowest. Conversely, when we're experiencing wakefulness, our core body temperature is at its highest. By paying attention to this body cue, we can figure out strategies to help us deal with certain situations.

With this in mind, there is a way to adapt our circadian rhythm timing.

On a podcast episode, Dr. Andrew Huberman mentioned using the concept of "temperature minimum" to realign circadian behavior during jet lag and shift work (Huberman, 2021a). This essentially refers to the time when our core body temperature is at its lowest in a 24-hour cycle. This often occurs roughly 90 minutes to two hours before our average wake-up time. The reason it's important is that body temperature is the key signal for setting circadian timing in all our organs and tissues. Temperature is the one thing that controls and coordinates all of our cells and neural circuitry to make us react in a predictable way. For instance, when our body is at its coldest temperature, it's time to facilitate sleep. Likewise, when our core body temperature hits its peak during the day, then it's time for us to be alert.

Note that our individual "temperature minimum" doesn't have to be measured in Fahrenheit. All we have to do is work out our average waking time and subtract roughly two hours from that. So, if we were to wake up at 7 a.m. typically, then our body's lowest temperature would be roughly 5 a.m. or 5:30 a.m. This is vital to know before delving into the following sections. Some of these strategies hinge on this factor, so it's best to figure it out beforehand.

As a result, we can use the idea of the "temperature minimum" as an anchor for our schedule. This happens by manipulating factors that stimulate our sleep-wake state around this time period. You guessed it, we can use the physiological cues of light, temperature, exercise, and timing of food intake to trick our bodies once again. By changing the environment at certain times of the day, we can create adaptive strategies that put us in the best possible state.

Social Jet Lag

So I want to address this type of jet-lagged state separately from travel jet lag since this one involves no change in time zone or location.

We experience social jet lag when the social timings of our obligations, such as work, school, etc., are drastically different from the biological timings of our circadian clocks and chronotypes. This is often caused by having two distinct sleeping patterns as opposed to a unified one; usually, it's split into a regular sleep schedule for weekdays and an altered sleep schedule for weekends.

But these two sleeping patterns can't coincide with one another without being detrimental to our health. It has been demonstrated that this nonstandard weekly schedule is not only impractical but also counterintuitive due to the constraints imposed on us by our social environments. While for some, it may be underlying health conditions causing these sleep irregularities, for many others, it's the result of shift work schedules and resisting our chronotypes.

This can negatively impact our health in a multitude of ways. By sleeping in later on the weekends, we are raising our stress levels, which inadvertently cause health risks linked to heart disease, type-2 diabetes, and obesity. Also, social jet lag makes it more likely that you'll feel sleepy during the day, have trouble falling asleep, and have other sleep problems like sleep apnea (Medic et al., 2017). This further exacerbates our emotional well-being, since we're probably disrupting the natural sleep architecture and not getting quality REM and slow-wave sleep.

Therefore, it actually becomes counterintuitive to get up early during the week and then have a sleep-in on the weekends. As I mentioned in the "Myths about Sleep" chapter, it's impossible to compensate for sleep debt. It's far better to focus on fine-tuning our lifestyle with the tools in this guidebook. Consistency is your friend here. As tempting as it can be, aim to keep a fixed sleeping pattern every day of the week. You'll want to wake up and go to sleep at the same time every day.

While it's difficult to maintain this balance, there is some leniency here. Thankfully, we can get away with a slightly altered sleep schedule as long as the difference doesn't exceed 30 minutes to an hour. This allows us some flexibility on the weekends if we really need it. Next, on your days off, please ensure that you maintain good sleep hygiene in your bedroom environment, utilize the tools of sunlight, exercise to great effect, and finally allow yourself power naps if the grogginess gets unbearable during the afternoons. By making this consistent daily effort, we can lessen the damage that social jet lag causes to our health.

Traveling Abroad

Travel jet lag is a serious issue that we've all undoubtedly faced. What many may not realize is that frequent jet lag has harmful effects that can shorten one's lifespan (Sack et al., 2007). Our brains are not designed to adjust to radical shifts in time zones and space. You may not need to worry about a large time difference if you're traveling northbound or southbound from your current location. Although, with that being said, it's far better for our health to travel westbound than eastbound across the globe. The latter is associated with a shorter life span of a few years (Davidson et al., 2006).

Since the tilt of the Earth's axis causes it to spin in a counterclockwise direction from west to east, this demonstrates that eastbound travel always has time zones ahead of our local schedule. Likewise, westbound travel has time zones behind our local schedule.

Now we need to consider this since our evolutionary conditioning is affected by it. A study showed how the life spans of people who traveled eastbound or westbound often were different from those who didn't travel at all. It turns out that our autonomic nervous systems are asymmetrically hardwired, meaning it is far easier for us to stay alert longer than to fall asleep earlier (Davidson et al., 2006). Therefore, when we travel eastbound, it can be difficult to fall asleep on the new local schedule since our circadian rhythms are still set to the old time schedule. This could mean that even though it's 2 a.m. in Tokyo, your body thinks it's 5 p.m. It should be clear now that westbound travel is easier to adjust to since we can prolong how long we stay awake and re-shift to the local schedule with less hassle.

Although avoiding jet lag can be difficult, it's not impossible.

Before going further, I want to point out that time zone jet lag and travel fatigue are mutually exclusive conditions. The first kind happens when our internal circadian rhythms aren't in sync with light and dark cues from the outside world. This makes us feel disoriented and confused about time and place. The latter is merely a general weariness felt when traveling internationally, north or south, and is a result of the lengthy travel experience, variations in air quality, etc. Travel fatigue is difficult to mitigate, but it tends to wear off eventually.

Additionally, if you're traveling for less than 72 hours, don't try to re-shift your circadian rhythm. Unfortunately, it can take up to two days for our circadian rhythms to adjust by a couple of hours. So it may not be worth employing the "temperature minimum" tactic in this case. Instead, if possible, try to reschedule meetings and appointments according to your normal time zone schedule. That way you can avoid dips in your performance during important work conversations with clients, colleagues, etc.

Now, if you're planning to travel for a longer period of time, say a week or so, then here are some guidelines to follow in the few days before you leave. To offset jet lag, we need to exploit the four- to six-hour time windows prior to and following the time when our bodies experience their lowest temperature. In this time frame, we're able to shift our body temperature, and this can have drastic effects on when our sleep-wake cycle is programmed.

For example, if you're traveling westbound, then take advantage of the four- to six-hour window before the time of your "temperature minimum". If you typically wake up at 6 a.m., then do this between 12 a.m. and 2 a.m. I know this sounds nuts, but it will work. What you want to do in this period is leverage the conditions that promote our typical physiological cues. That's right, you want to expose yourself to light (artificial lighting is fine here) and raise your core temperature through exercise and/or a cold bath, as well as consume some food and drink.

By manipulating these factors, you will cause what is known as a "phase delay" in your circadian clock (Sack et al., 2007). This simply means that your body temperature has risen out of sync, and it takes longer for it to drop back and dip to its lowest level in a 24-hour interval. Hence, your body temperature will be raised higher later in the day than normal, and this will inevitably make you stay awake longer, helping you to adjust to the new time zone you'll soon be in.

Conversely, if you're traveling eastbound, then you want to do the exact opposite of what I recommended. In this case, you'll take advantage of the four- to six-hour window after the time of your "temperature minimum." So, if you wake up at 6 a.m., then manipulate those aforementioned factors between 10 a.m. and 12 p.m. Again, at these times, expose yourself to appropriate lighting, exercise, and/or that cold bath, as well as eat and drink something. By raising your body temperature at this time, you will cause your circadian clock to experience a "phase advance" in its timing. As your body temperature soars, it will fall quicker by the evening. Therefore, it will make you fall asleep earlier in the day and you'll quickly adjust to the new time zone you'll soon be in.

Now, there are some handy tricks to maintain this

strategy before and during your trip. To keep accurate track of the time, perhaps set the new time zone of your destination on your watch or phone. This will not only help you monitor the time of your typical "thermal minimum," but it'll also help you predict when you should be alert and when you should be asleep. Wearable digital tools (Fitbit, Oura, and Whoop) that can monitor your body temperature are also useful for checking in on whether or not you've successfully adjusted your circadian rhythm. Especially use these devices when you arrive abroad, since they will collectively ensure that you phase-shift your circadian rhythm consistently. Finally, try to time your schedule according to the local time zone. For example, you will want to eat when the locals eat their meals. This will ensure that the biological clocks in your organs and tissues respond to this new time zone appropriately.

Shift Work

Let me start by saying that shift work is essential in our modern age. The type of work I'm referring to involves working flexible, odd hours, either at home or in the workplace, that help ensure smooth day-to-day operations in our society. Whether it's working on laptops or computers, emergency response, healthcare, hospitality, warehouse distribution, or many other work sectors, it's virtually impossible for our society to function without the tremendous dedication of shift workers.

That being said, the importance of shift work sadly doesn't negate the severe health implications it raises. We've already discussed issues related to compromised immunity and the development of conditions such as shift work sleep disorder (SWSD), but there are methods to mitigate these issues that can flare up in our shift-work lifestyle.

The first tactic involves trying to negotiate with your boss to work a fixed schedule for at least a fortnight. This allows you to at least control the underlying behavioral tools that influence the sleep-wake state and overall helps you establish a consistent rhythm in your 24-hour schedule. However, this may not even be remotely possible for many of us who are shift workers.

The second-best option is to leverage these tools according to your schedule. For example, night shift workers operate on an inverted schedule compared to those who work during the day. Therefore, it makes practical sense to take advantage of nocturnal habits as opposed to strictly following them in a diurnal manner. Let's assume you wake up as the sun sets in the evening. This would be your typical wake-up cue to begin the day, and thus you'd follow the tools in the "Perfect Your Morning" chapter. This is a circumstance where it's already dark outside, so you'd manipulate artificial light in the form of sun lamps or light therapy boxes while also relying on the cues from overhead lighting.

As the night shift progresses, you keep leveraging this light tool, ensuring you view some form of light during your working hours so you can maintain alertness. Additionally, you'd use the tools to help maintain a productive day wherever it is possible. When your shift finally ends, you want to begin the process of winding down. This involves the tools outlined in "Fall Asleep Like a Pro," where you'd want to simmer down and avoid viewing light as much as possible. Since night shift workers have an adapted circadian rhythm that is timed under inverted conditions, the sunrise actually becomes the cue to wind down.

But what happens the following day? Well, this is where the tool of "temperature minimum" comes into play once again. You want to monitor this physiological cue whenever you wake up. If you feel cold, then don't view the light, but if you feel warm, then view the light. The time you wake up doesn't matter here—it's more about your internal rhythm state. If we can pinpoint our core body temperature, we can figure out when we need to maintain wakefulness or induce sleepiness.

On that note, we can carefully time our meals so they naturally realign our circadian rhythm. Studies have shown that our daytime eating habits set the biological clocks in our organs, helping us to maintain glucose levels within normal ranges (Wehrens et al., 2017). Therefore, this can help us when we do night shift work: by eating earlier in the day, we can reduce blood spikes and dips in energy, and ultimately maintain alertness during night working hours. This behavior weaves nicely into our inverted circadian rhythm, allowing us to fall asleep after a long night shift without the added burden of a stuffed stomach.

Eventually, we'll develop a consistent circadian rhythm that makes intuitive sense for our schedule.

However, I realize that this adaptive strategy may seem unconventional. It will certainly be difficult for those who have to take care of families after work. This isn't to say that you must neglect your responsibilities, but rather that you should adopt an approach that helps you balance your health and relationships appropriately. Flexible work hours can be very hard on your health, so it's important for shift workers to develop a regular internal rhythm. So, I suggest that you use this toolkit to find a way to adapt to your situation so that your sleep doesn't suffer for no reason.

Parenthood

This is a section for expecting parents or those navigating the challenges of new parenthood. It's no secret that parents suffer from sleep deprivation during the early stages of childhood.

Needless to say, parents drastically lose thousands of hours of sleep over the course of infanthood. Especially mothers, who are more likely to have trouble sleeping because of all the stress that comes with being a parent at night (CDC, 2019). A 2004 study highlighted that this sleep deprivation can be prolonged over at least the first six years of early childhood (Gay et al., 2004). Also, an imbalance in hormone levels can make it hard to sleep as a parent, especially for women whose estrogen and progesterone levels drop after giving birth. As a result, this makes whatever amount of shut-eye you get far less restorative in the process. We already know how this can greatly impact stress levels and increase the risk of underlying health issues in the long term.

However, that isn't to say that only a bleak outcome lies on the horizon.

While we'll hear the baby's cries in the middle of the night and reluctantly tend to feedings, changing diapers, and everything else that goes with early child rearing, it doesn't mean we have to completely neglect our sleep hygiene. During this turbulent time, it's critical to manage our own health to avoid major issues like general irritability, mental illness, and accidents caused by self-neglect and accumulated exhaustion.

Again, we can adapt a strategy using the toolkit highlighted throughout this book.

Babies have reduced sleep cycles, sleeping a mere one to three hours before they inevitably wake up. This is because an infant hasn't developed any sense of circadian rhythm yet, so their timing is naturally out of sync. As a result, it affects their eating patterns as well as their sleeping habits.

Since babies don't sleep at the same time every night, we can use naps to great effect. Use this invaluable tool when the baby is sleeping: whenever the baby naps, you should nap as well. In particular, parents can use a polyphasic sleep schedule to their advantage. This is when a person sleeps at different times of the day for shorter amounts of time. While it sounds daunting, this polyphasic sleep is flexible for any routine and has various methods and timeframes that can be adopted by anyone. Though these short bouts only give you a brief window of rest, they will still provide a remarkable boost in energy on turbulent days.

So, parenthood is the exception to the rule: use the napping tool as often as you'd like.

Similarly, you should improve your sleep hygiene by developing a bedtime routine and creating an ideal sleep environment in both your and your child's bedrooms. It is especially important to create a nighttime ritual involving your child, like reading them a story under a dim light setting, so you craft a natural wind-down cue in their surrounding environment. When it comes to your own environment, remember that your bedroom has to be cool, dark, and quiet to optimize sleep. Now, this obviously won't guarantee fewer nighttime wakings, but it'll help ease the burden significantly.

Next, if you share parenting duties with someone, you should both communicate and plan a functional schedule together. This involves having one person delegated to take over the night watch duties for a night while the other person sleeps. A coordinated effort like this can ensure that you both have at least a good night's rest every other day. So, the person who gets to rest can either sleep in a separate bedroom or use an eye mask and earplugs to help them rest well.

Aside from that, you should set clear boundaries when it comes to families and friends. Don't be afraid to say no to their visits or even delay them so you can adjust comfortably into a settled routine with your child. That being said, it's also vital to ask for help whenever you need it. While you can rely on your partner for assistance, you may also need additional help from others. Don't be afraid to delegate responsibilities to those who can help, so you can take time to recuperate and focus on your own health needs.

Finally, the last thing you may want to consider is sleep training. Although we shouldn't recklessly dismiss nighttime wakings, there are infant sleep training routines that parents can do after the first six months of infancy. This is difficult to do, as it involves several methods that condition the baby's response when they cry in the middle of the night. If possible, you can try to let them cry it out and not respond to it, so the behavior gets extinguished.

Harsh, I know.

Other alternatives include Ferber's controlled crying method, where you gradually ignore their cries over longer periods of time (Breus, 2022); the camping-out method, where a parent stays present in the room all night but doesn't respond to the crying (Breus, 2022); bedtime fading, where you gradually put the child to sleep earlier or later until you reach the ideal bedtime schedule (Gradisar et al., 2016); and finally, there are scheduled awakenings, where you preemptively wake up the baby the night before they're scheduled to be awake and soothe them (Breus, 2022). While these methods have shown proven results, they also disrupt the parent's sleeping schedule, which could do more harm than good. Then again, they can also alleviate the parental burden and reduce sleep deprivation, along with the host of maladies that tag along with it.

Overall, I hope that some of these strategies prove useful to your circumstances, regardless of which stage of parenthood you're currently navigating.

Tool 14: Supplements to Fortify Your Rest

Even with all the tools provided so far, it's important to discuss supplements. Nature has provided essential nutrients for the human brain and body, yet even with a balanced diet, it can be difficult to get the recommended dosages from food alone. In this section, I'll specifically highlight the benefits of these sleep nutrients, their dietary sources, and how to supplement your lifestyle with their manufactured forms as well.

I want to preface this section with the following note: These supplements should not be taken instead of following the prescribed tools to hack your sleep. Treat them as an aid to boosting the chance of success. I recommend that you try to get these nutrients from their natural food sources first, if you can, before you look into the recommended supplement dose.

Magnesium

This is an important mineral that helps regulate a lot of diverse mechanisms in the body. For instance, it not only maintains brain function and heart health but also significantly contributes to improving sleep. It has a relaxation effect on muscles by stimulating melatonin production and also increases inhibitory neurotransmitter levels, such as GABA. This combined effect helps facilitate the onset of sleep and improves sleep quality.

We can find good sources of magnesium naturally in our diet by consuming nuts, seeds, leafy green vegetables, legumes, and whole grains. As for the recommended dietary intake, it's advisable not to exceed 350 mg per day (Frank et al., 2019).

If you opt to take the supplement form, magnesium is best taken 30 to 60 minutes before bed. However, there is a way to enhance the relaxing effects of this vital mineral. When paired with the amino acid glycine to form magnesium glycinate, this supplement can have substantial calming effects on the body. Glycine is an inhibitory neurotransmitter like GABA. It helps fight free radicals and lowers the body's core temperature, which can help you fall asleep.

L-Ornithine

Although this isn't an essential amino acid, it's an important one that actually improves athletic performance. But I recommend it in this section because it can help reduce anxiety, speed up physical recovery, and keep the liver working well.

This nutrient gives a supplementary boost to growth hormone production and hence reduces general fatigue while improving cardiovascular function and muscle repair. Studies have also shown that l-ornithine makes people less tired by easing stress and making them sleep better (Miyake et al., 2014; Takakura et al., 2022).

There are good levels of l-ornithine in high-protein sources like eggs, red meat, poultry, fish, and dairy. In supplement form, taking 1.5 g of l-ornithine should suffice (Patel, 2022).

Ashwagandha

This is a shrub that grows natively in parts of Asia and Africa, and it's often used for its stress-relieving benefits. Ashwagandha, or "winter cherry," as it's commonly known, mediates the stress response in our bodies by influencing components involved in the physiological mechanism. For instance, this adaptogen can regulate cortisol and other pathway proteins and also reduce activity in parts of the autonomic nervous system.

Ashwagandha also has antidepressant properties, increases testosterone and fertility, and lowers blood sugar levels and inflammation. Needless to say, it also contributes to improved sleep quality, which is why it's included on this list.

Ashwagandha root can be supplemented in pill, powder, or liquid form, and the dosages for this can vary from 250 mg to 2 g (Frank et al., 2020). If you're taking it as a powder or liquid, it's often mixed into drinks and served with a meal. Please note that the health benefits of this supplement can take up to a month to take effect. So be patient and consistent when using it.

Rhodiola

This is a flower that naturally grows in arctic regions of Asia, Europe, and parts of North America. Its root is considered a stress antigen, having similar calming effects to ashwagandha. Notably, rhodiola relieves burnout symptoms provoked by chronic stress and even alleviates fatigue.

A possible reason for this is that some studies

demonstrate that flowers aid in physical and mental performance and also boost concentration. Some studies even showed rhodiola's anxiety-relieving effects as well (Frank et al., 2021).

Again, this flower is commonly sourced in capsule, liquid, or powder form. The recommended dosage is 100mg to 6 mg (Frank et al., 2021). It's important to note that rhodiola has energizing properties, while ashwagandha has soothing properties. So, to get the most health benefits from this supplement, it's best to take it early in the day.

Conclusion

Overall, I think that these supplements will provide that extra edge throughout your day. Use them sparingly at different times in your routine. By paying attention to our nutritional habits, we can influence their dynamic relationship with our sleep. Therefore, we can revitalize our energy and performance but also urge ourselves into a restful slumber at the end of the day.

While we struggle to keep up with the demands of a fast-paced world, we can still leverage this toolkit to great effect. This chapter has shown irrefutable proof of this. All of the basic tools in this book can be used to make plans that, in the end, have a big impact on our biology. I hope that by sharing this knowledge, I've eliminated the overwhelming process of trial and error.

We don't have to needlessly surrender to weariness. Whether we're struggling to balance night shift work and parenthood or we're suffering from prolonged bouts of social and travel jet lag, we can use the science of our bodies to make life easier. The integral nature of these mechanisms that keep us awake and help us fall asleep all exist in harmony. Amidst the chaos of 21st-century living, we can restore balance by being intuitively aware of the physiological cues influencing us.

In general, we should pay attention to our environment and observe how it affects our individual bodies. Specifically, we should figure out our chronotypes through self-assessment; this gives us the advantage of optimizing performance every single day. For the most part, use the flexible toolkit in this book to suit your individual circumstances. In whatever situation arises in our day-to-day lives, we can comfortably adapt these strategies and leverage them to great effect.

Final Thoughts

Do you see how the pieces of the puzzle finally fit together?

The enigmatic nature of sleep has finally been unraveled. Throughout the book, I've highlighted the mechanisms involved in our sleep-wake state that govern our day-to-day lives. It is from this new insight that we can garner flexibility in our lifestyle and make intuitive decisions that make sense for us.

Now that you've reached the end of this guidebook, I hope that I've shed some insight into sleep's scientific blueprint. It's important for me to share this knowledge and promote better sleeping habits and behaviors to help re-educate the public.

By changing our routines with the help of this toolkit, we can get the most out of our sleep and feel more refreshed. In the first section of the book, I highlight the remarkable skill of sleeping and the tremendous health benefits it provides to every aspect of our health. Together, we've explored the circadian and chemical forces underlying our sleep-wake state and all the unified effort that goes into coordinating the timing of our sleep rhythm during a typical day.

From there, I've laid out behavioral guidelines that can be followed daily. Every practical tool and strategy has been backed up with the latest scientific evidence. They can all be stacked together or uniquely tailored to your individualized experience. I've laid them out in a straightforward manner so you, the reader, can leverage them in your mornings, afternoons, and evenings to maximum effect.

Finally, I've discussed how to deal with sleep issues in the modern world. Particularly, the frustrations of sleep interruptions: all those middle-of-the-night excursions, mind-wandering tours, and sleepless woes. We've looked at adaptive strategies that deal with chronotypes, jet lag, sleep debt, working shifts, and even being a parent. I then briefly broached the topic of supplementation and how we can use certain nutrients to fortify our sleep quality and duration. While these tactics may not create the ideal conditions for sleeping, they will at least mitigate the impact of sleep deprivation on our health and longevity.

But even with all the information in this guidebook, in the end, you must be responsible for your own health. I firmly believe that if you apply one or more of the prescribed tools outlined here, you're taking a stride in the right direction for your well-being. After all, it's about the return on investment. If you commit to these long-term habits and behaviors, you can increase your maximum energy and perform at your best.

Who wouldn't want to live a more revitalized lifestyle?

Ultimately, this guidebook is about fixing irregularities in our sleeping patterns. In this fast-paced modern age we live in, we need to prioritize self-care now more than ever before. It's important to point out that as you adopt these tools into your daily routine, it will take time to notice adjustments in your sleep.

Treat each day as an incremental step toward your end goal of better sleep. Your plan to improve your performance and liven up your life will eventually come to fruition. We don't need to aim for perfection when using this toolkit. If we break a habit one day, it doesn't undo all the hard work we've done so far. It is only through the practice of consistency that you'll truly notice marked improvement in your overall health and well-being.

By following the tools and strategies in this book, you will transform the quality of your life: it will be enriched with an abundance of energy, ease, and joy. After all, science will certainly guarantee it.

References

Alhola, P., & Polo-Kantola, P. (2007). Sleep deprivation: Impact on cognitive performance. Neuropsychiatric Disease and Treatment, 3(5), 553–567.

Alley, J. R., Mazzochi, J. W., Smith, C. J., Morris, D. M., & Collier, S. R. (2015). Effects of Resistance Exercise Timing on Sleep Architecture and Nocturnal Blood Pressure. Journal of Strength and Conditioning Research, 29(5), 1378–1385. https://doi.org/10.1519/jsc.0000000000000750

Almutawa, F., Vandal, R., Wang, S. Q., & Lim, H. W. (2013). Current status of photoprotection by window glass, automobile glass, window films, and sunglasses. Photodermatology, Photoimmunology & Photomedicine, 29(2), 65–72. https://doi.org/10.1111/phpp.12022

Andreani, T. S., Itoh, T. Q., Yildirim, E., Hwangbo, D.-S., & Allada, R. (2015). Genetics of Circadian Rhythms. Sleep Medicine Clinics, 10(4), 413–421. https://doi.org/10.1016/j.jsmc.2015.08.007

Arain, M., Mathur, P., Rais, A., Nel, W., Sandhu, R., Haque, M., Johal, L., & Sharma, S. (2013). Maturation of the Adolescent Brain. Neuropsychiatric Disease and Treatment, 9(9), 449–461. https://doi.org/10.2147/ndt.s39776

Avidan, A., & Colwell, C. (2010). Jet lag syndrome: circadian organization, pathophysiology, and management strategies. Nature and Science of Sleep, 2, 187. https://doi.org/10.2147/nss.s6683

Battistella, G., Fornari, E., Annoni, J.-M., Chtioui, H., Dao, K., Fabritius, M., Favrat, B., Mall, J.-F., Maeder, P., & Giroud, C. (2014). Long-Term Effects of Cannabis on Brain Structure. Neuropsychopharmacology, 39(9), 2041–2048. https://doi.org/10.1038/npp.2014.67

Beaulieu, K., Oustric, P., Alkahtani, S., Alhussain, M., Pedersen, H., Salling Quist, J., Færch, K., & Finlayson, G. (2020). Impact of Meal Timing and Chronotype on Food Reward and Appetite Control in Young Adults. Nutrients, 12(5), 1506. https://doi.org/10.3390/nu12051506

Benz, A., Meier, M., Mankin, M., Unternaehrer, E., & Pruessner, J. C. (2019). The duration of the cortisol awakening pulse exceeds sixty minutes in a meaningful pattern. Psychoneuroendocrinology, 105, 187–194. https://doi.org/10.1016/j.psyneuen.2018.12.225

Berger, M., Gray, J. A., & Roth, B. L. (2009). The expanded biology of serotonin. Annual Review of Medicine, 60(1), 355–366. https://doi.org/10.1146/annurev.med.60.042307.110802

Besedovsky, L., Lange, T., & Born, J. (2011). Sleep and immune function. Pflügers Archiv - European Journal of Physiology, 463(1), 121–137. https://doi.org/10.1007/s00424-011-1044-0

Bjorness, T. E., & Greene, R. W. (2009). Adenosine and Sleep. Current Neuropharmacology, 7(3), 238–245. https://doi.org/10.2174/157015909789152182

Blume, C., Garbazza, C., & Spitschan, M. (2019). Effects of light on human circadian rhythms, sleep and mood. Somnologie : Schlafforschung Und Schlafmedizin = Somnology : Sleep Research and Sleep Medicine, 23(3), 147–156. https://doi.org/10.1007/s11818-019-00215-x

Bonora, M., Patergnani, S., Rimessi, A., De Marchi, E., Suski, J. M., Bononi, A., Giorgi, C., Marchi, S., Missiroli, S., Poletti, F., Wieckowski, M. R., & Pinton, P. (2012). ATP synthesis and storage. Purinergic Signalling, 8(3), 343–357. https://doi.org/10.1007/s11302-012-9305-8

Borea, P. A., Gessi, S., Merighi, S., Vincenzi, F., & Varani, K. (2017). Pathological overproduction: the bad side of adenosine. British Journal of Pharmacology, 174(13), 1945–1960. https://doi.org/10.1111/bph.13763

Boukhris, O., Trabelsi, K., Ammar, A., Abdessalem, R., Hsouna, H., Glenn, J. M., Bott, N., Driss, T., Souissi, N., Hammouda, O., Garbarino, S., Bragazzi, N. L., & Chtourou, H. (2020). A 90 min Daytime Nap Opportunity Is Better Than 40 min for Cognitive and Physical Performance. International Journal of Environmental Research and Public Health, 17(13), 4650. https://doi.org/10.3390/ijerph17134650

Boyon, N. (2022). Global Happiness 2022: what makes people happy in the age of COVID-19.In https://

www.ipsos.com/en/global-happiness-survey-march-2022 (pp.13–16).Ipsos. https://www.ipsos.com/sites/default/files/ct/news/documents/2022-04/Global%20Happiness%202022%20Report.pdf

Branzei, D., & Foiani, M. (2008). Regulation of DNA repair throughout the cell cycle. Nature Reviews Molecular Cell Biology, 9(4), 297–308. https://doi.org/10.1038/nrm2351

Breus, D. M. (2022, September 8). How to Sleep Train Babies. The Sleep Doctor. https://thesleepdoctor.com/baby-sleep/sleep-training/

Brinkman, J. E., Tariq, M. A., Leavitt, L., & Sharma, S. (2022). Physiology, Growth Hormone. In StatPearls. StatPearls Publishing; StatPearls. https://www.ncbi.nlm.nih.gov/books/NBK482141/

Brooks, A., & Lack, L. (2006). A Brief Afternoon Nap Following Nocturnal Sleep Restriction: Which Nap Duration is Most Recuperative? Sleep, 29(6), 831–840. https://doi.org/10.1093/sleep/29.6.831

Brown, T. M., Brainard, G. C., Cajochen, C., Czeisler, C. A., Hanifin, J. P., Lockley, S. W., Lucas, R. J., Münch, M., O'Hagan, J. B., Peirson, S. N., Price, L. L. A., Roenneberg, T., Schlangen, L. J. M., Skene, D. J., Spitschan, M., Vetter, C., Zee, P. C., & Wright, K. P. (2022). Recommendations for daytime, evening, and nighttime indoor light exposure to best support physiology, sleep, and wakefulness in healthy adults. PLOS Biology, 20(3), e3001571. https://doi.org/10.1371/journal.pbio.3001571

Buhr, E. D., Yoo, S.-H. ., & Takahashi, J. S. (2010). Temperature as a Universal Resetting Cue for Mammalian Circadian Oscillators. Science, 330(6002), 379–385. https://doi.org/10.1126/science.1195262

Burgess, H. J., & Molina, T. A. (2014). Home lighting before usual bedtime impacts circadian timing: a field study. Photochemistry and Photobiology, 90(3), 723–726. https://doi.org/10.1111/php.12241

Caliandro, R., Streng, A. A., van Kerkhof, L. W. M., van der Horst, G. T. J., & Chaves, I. (2021). Social Jetlag and Related Risks for Human Health: A Timely Review. Nutrients, 13(12), 4543. https://doi.org/10.3390/nu13124543

CDC. (2017). CDC - How Much Sleep Do I Need? - Sleep and Sleep Disorders. CDC; CDC. https://www.cdc.gov/sleep/about_sleep/how_much_sleep.html

CDC. (2019). Depression Among Women. Centers for Disease Control and Prevention. https://www.cdc.gov/reproductivehealth/depression/index.htm

Cederbaum, A. I. (2012). Alcohol Metabolism. Clinics in Liver Disease, 16(4), 667–685. https://doi.org/10.1016/j.cld.2012.08.002

Chang, A.-M., Aeschbach, D., Duffy, J. F., & Czeisler, C. A. (2014). Evening use of light-emitting eReaders negatively affects sleep, circadian timing, and next-morning alertness. Proceedings of the National Academy of Sciences, 112(4), 1232–1237. https://

doi.org/10.1073/pnas.1418490112

Chaput, J.-P., Dutil, C., Featherstone, R., Ross, R., Giangregorio, L., Saunders, T. J., Janssen, I., Poitras, V. J., Kho, M. E., Ross-White, A., Zankar, S., & Carrier, J. (2020). Sleep timing, sleep consistency, and health in adults: a systematic review. Applied Physiology, Nutrition, and Metabolism, 45(10 (Suppl. 2)), S232–S247. https://doi.org/10.1139/apnm-2020-0032

Chattu, V., Manzar, Md., Kumary, S., Burman, D., Spence, D., & Pandi-Perumal, S. (2018). The Global Problem of Insufficient Sleep and Its Serious Public Health Implications. Healthcare, 7(1), 1. NCBI. https://doi.org/10.3390/healthcare7010001

Chellappa, S. L., Qian, J., Vujovic, N., Morris, C. J., Nedeltcheva, A., Nguyen, H., Rahman, N., Heng, S. W., Kelly, L., Kerlin-Monteiro, K., Srivastav, S., Wang, W., Aeschbach, D., Czeisler, C. A., Shea, S. A., Adler, G. K., Garaulet, M., & Scheer, F. A. J. L. (2021). Daytime eating prevents internal circadian misalignment and glucose intolerance in night work. Science Advances, 7(49). https://doi.org/10.1126/sciadv.abg9910

Collier, S., Fairbrother, K., Cartner, B., Alley, J., Curry, C., Dickinson, D., & Morris, D. (2014). Effects of exercise timing on sleep architecture and nocturnal blood pressure in prehypertensives. Vascular Health and Risk Management, 691. https://doi.org/10.2147/vhrm.s73688

Colrain, I. M., Nicholas, C. L., & Baker, F. C. (2014). Alcohol and the sleeping brain. Handbook of Clinical Neurology, 125, 415–431. https://doi.org/10.1016/b978-0-444-62619-6.00024-0

Colten, H. R., & Altevogt, B. M. (Eds.). (2006a). Extent and Health Consequences of Chronic Sleep Loss and Sleep Disorders. In Sleep disorders and sleep deprivation : an unmet public health problem. National Academy of Sciences.

Colten, H. R., & Altevogt, B. M. (Eds.). (2006b). Sleep Physiology. In Sleep disorders and sleep deprivation : an unmet public health problem. National Academy of Sciences.

Dagnino-Subiabre, A., Orellana, J. A., Carmona-Fontaine, C., Montiel, J., Diaz-Veliz, G., Seron-Ferre, M., Wyneken, U., Concha, M. L., & Aboitiz, F. (2006). Chronic stress decreases the expression of sympathetic markers in the pineal gland and increases plasma melatonin concentration in rats. Journal of Neurochemistry, 97(5), 1279–1287. https://doi.org/10.1111/j.1471-4159.2006.03787.x

Datta, K., Tripathi, M., Verma, M., Masiwal, D., & Mallick, H. N. (2021). Yoga nidra practice shows improvement in sleep in patients with chronic insomnia: A randomized controlled trial. The National Medical Journal of India, 34, 143–150. https://doi.org/10.25259/nmji_63_19

Dattilo, M., Antunes, H. K. M., Medeiros, A., Mônico Neto, M., Souza, H. S., Tufik, S., & de Mello, M. T. (2011). Sleep and muscle recovery: Endocrinological and molecular basis for a new and promising hypothesis. Medical Hypotheses, 77(2), 220–222. https://doi.org/10.1016/j.mehy.2011.04.017

Davidson, A., Sellix, M., Daniel, J., Yamazaki, S., Menaker, M., & Block, G. (2006). Chronic jet-lag increases mortality in aged mice. Current Biology : CB, 16(21), R914–R916. https://doi.org/10.1016/j.cub.2006.09.058

Del Bene, V. E. (1990). Temperature. In Clinical methods : the history, physical and laboratory examinations (3rd ed.). Butterworths. https://www.ncbi.nlm.nih.gov/books/NBK201/

De Lorenzo, B. H. P., de Oliveira Marchioro, L., Greco, C. R., & Suchecki, D. (2015). Sleep-deprivation reduces NK cell number and function mediated by β-adrenergic signalling. Psychoneuroendocrinology, 57, 134–143. https://doi.org/10.1016/j.psyneuen.2015.04.006

Dolezal, B. A., Neufeld, E. V., Boland, D. M., Martin, J. L., & Cooper, C. B. (2017). Interrelationship between Sleep and Exercise: a Systematic Review. Advances in Preventive Medicine, 2017(1364387), 1–14. https://doi.org/10.1155/2017/1364387

Eban-Rothschild, A., Appelbaum, L., & de Lecea, L. (2018). Neuronal Mechanisms for Sleep/Wake Regulation and Modulatory Drive. Neuropsychopharmacology, 43(5), 937–952. https://doi.org/10.1038/npp.2017.294

F. Duffy, J., Scheuermaier, K., & R. Loughlin, K. (2015).

Age-Related Sleep Disruption and Reduction in the Circadian Rhythm of Urine Output: Contribution to Nocturia? Current Aging Science, 9(1), 34–43. https://doi.org/10.2174/1874609809666151130220343

Fischer, D., Lombardi, D. A., Marucci-Wellman, H., & Roenneberg, T. (2017). Chronotypes in the US – Influence of age and sex. PLOS ONE, 12(6), e0178782. https://doi.org/10.1371/journal.pone.0178782

Frank, K., Patel, K., Lopez, G., & Willis, B. (2019). Magnesium Research Analysis. Examine.com. https://examine.com/supplements/magnesium/

Frank, K., Patel, K., Lopez, G., & Willis, B. (2020). Ashwagandha Research Analysis. Examine.com. https://examine.com/supplements/ashwagandha/

Frank, K., Patel, K., Lopez, G., & Willis, B. (2021). Rhodiola Rosea Research Analysis. Examine.com. https://examine.com/supplements/rhodiola-rosea/

Fujiwara, Y., Arakawa, T., & Fass, R. (2012). Gastroesophageal reflux disease and sleep disturbances. Journal of Gastroenterology, 47(7), 760–769. https://doi.org/10.1007/s00535-012-0601-4

Gandhi, Avni V., Mosser, E. A., Oikonomou, G., & Prober, David A. (2015). Melatonin Is Required for the Circadian Regulation of Sleep. Neuron, 85(6), 1193–1199. https://doi.org/10.1016/j.neuron.2015.02.016

Gay, C. L., Lee, K. A., & Lee, S.-Y. (2004). Sleep Patterns

and Fatigue in New Mothers and Fathers. Biological Research for Nursing, 5(4), 311–318. https://doi.org/10.1177/1099800403262142

Gilbert, S. S., van den Heuvel, C. J., Ferguson, S. A., & Dawson, D. (2004). Thermoregulation as a sleep signalling system. Sleep Medicine Reviews, 8(2), 81–93. https://doi.org/10.1016/S1087-0792(03)00023-6

Ginta, D., & Grant, C. S. (2021, January 4). The tips and uses for magnesium glycinate. Healthline. https://www.healthline.com/health/magnesium-glycinate

Goldstein, A. N., Greer, S. M., Saletin, J. M., Harvey, A. G., Nitschke, J. B., & Walker, M. P. (2013). Tired and Apprehensive: Anxiety Amplifies the Impact of Sleep Loss on Aversive Brain Anticipation. Journal of Neuroscience, 33(26), 10607–10615. https://doi.org/10.1523/jneurosci.5578-12.2013

Gotter, A. (2018, January 11). Shift Work Sleep Disorder: Treatment, Diagnosis, Disability, and More. Healthline. https://www.healthline.com/health/shift-work-sleep-disorder#lifestyle-changes

Gradisar, M., Jackson, K., Spurrier, N. J., Gibson, J., Whitham, J., Williams, A. S., Dolby, R., & Kennaway, D. J. (2016). Behavioral Interventions for Infant Sleep Problems: A Randomized Controlled Trial. Pediatrics, 137(6), e20151486–e20151486. https://doi.org/10.1542/peds.2015-1486

Grandner, M. A., Jackson, N., Gerstner, J. R., & Knutson,

K. L. (2013). Sleep symptoms associated with intake of specific dietary nutrients. Journal of Sleep Research, 23(1), 22–34. https://doi.org/10.1111/jsr.12084

Grant, C. L., Dorrian, J., Coates, A. M., Pajcin, M., Kennaway, D. J., Wittert, G. A., Heilbronn, L. K., Vedova, C. D., Gupta, C. C., & Banks, S. (2017). The impact of meal timing on performance, sleepiness, gastric upset, and hunger during simulated night shift. Industrial Health, 55(5), 423–436. https://doi.org/10.2486/indhealth.2017-0047

Haghayegh, S., Khoshnevis, S., Smolensky, M. H., Diller, K. R., & Castriotta, R. J. (2019). Before-bedtime passive body heating by warm shower or bath to improve sleep: A systematic review and meta-analysis. Sleep Medicine Reviews, 46, 124–135. https://doi.org/10.1016/j.smrv.2019.04.008

Hallegraeff, J. M., van der Schans, C. P., de Ruiter, R., & de Greef, M. H. G. (2012). Stretching before sleep reduces the frequency and severity of nocturnal leg cramps in older adults: a randomised trial. Journal of Physiotherapy, 58(1), 17–22. https://doi.org/10.1016/S1836-9553(12)70068-1

Hamilton, N. A., Nelson, C. A., Stevens, N., & Kitzman, H. (2006). Sleep and psychological well-being. Social Indicators Research, 82(1), 147–163. https://doi.org/10.1007/s11205-006-9030-1

Harding, E. C., Franks, N. P., & Wisden, W. (2019). The Temperature Dependence of Sleep. Frontiers in

Neuroscience, 13. https://doi.org/10.3389/fnins.2019.00336

Harding, E. C., Franks, N. P., & Wisden, W. (2020). Sleep and thermoregulation. Current Opinion in Physiology, 15, 7–13. https://doi.org/10.1016/j.cophys.2019.11.008

Harvard School Of Public Health. (2020, July 30). Caffeine. The Nutrition Source. https://www.hsph.harvard.edu/nutritionsource/caffeine/

Harvey, A. G., & Payne, S. (2002). The management of unwanted pre-sleep thoughts in insomnia: distraction with imagery versus general distraction. Behaviour Research and Therapy, 40(3), 267–277. https://doi.org/10.1016/s0005-7967(01)00012-2

Hattar, S. (2002). Melanopsin-Containing Retinal Ganglion Cells: Architecture, Projections, and Intrinsic Photosensitivity. Science, 295(5557), 1065–1070. https://doi.org/10.1126/science.1069609

Hilditch, C. J., Centofanti, S. A., Dorrian, J., & Banks, S. (2016). A 30-Minute, but Not a 10-Minute Nighttime Nap is Associated with Sleep Inertia. Sleep, 39(3), 675–685. https://doi.org/10.5665/sleep.5550

Hilditch, C. J., Dorrian, J., & Banks, S. (2016). Time to wake up: reactive countermeasures to sleep inertia. Industrial Health, 54(6), 528–541. https://doi.org/10.2486/indhealth.2015-0236

Hilditch, C. J., Dorrian, J., & Banks, S. (2017). A review of short naps and sleep inertia: do naps of 30 min or less really avoid sleep inertia and slow-wave sleep? Sleep Medicine, 32, 176–190. https://doi.org/10.1016/j.sleep.2016.12.016

Hill, V. M., O'Connor, R. M., Sissoko, G. B., Irobunda, I. S., Leong, S., Canman, J. C., Stavropoulos, N., & Shirasu-Hiza, M. (2018). A bidirectional relationship between sleep and oxidative stress in Drosophila. PLOS Biology, 16(7), e2005206. https://doi.org/10.1371/journal.pbio.2005206

Hiscock, H., Bayer, J., Gold, L., Hampton, A., Ukoumunne, O. C., & Wake, M. (2007). Improving infant sleep and maternal mental health: a cluster randomised trial. Archives of Disease in Childhood, 92(11), 952–958. https://doi.org/10.1136/adc.2006.099812

Holzman, D. C. (2010). What's in a Color? The Unique Human Health Effects of Blue Light. Environmental Health Perspectives, 118(1). https://doi.org/10.1289/ehp.118-a22

Huberman, A. (2021a). Find Your Temperature Minimum to Defeat Jetlag, Shift Work & Sleeplessness | Huberman Lab Podcast #4. In YouTube. https://www.youtube.com/watch?v=NAATB55oxeQ

Huberman, A. (2021b). Dr. Matthew Walker: The Science & Practice of Perfecting Your Sleep | Huberman Lab Podcast #31. In YouTube. https://www.youtube.com/watch?v=gbQFSMayJxk

IARC Working Group on the Identification of Carcinogenic Hazards to Humans. (2020). Night shift work: IARC Monographs on the Identification of Carcinogenic Hazards to Humans (Vol. 124, pp. 1–371). International Agency For Research On Cancer, World Health Organization.

Ibarra-Coronado, E. G., Pantaleón-Martínez, A. Ma., Velazquéz-Moctezuma, J., Prospéro-García, O., Méndez-Díaz, M., Pérez-Tapia, M., Pavón, L., & Morales-Montor, J. (2015). The Bidirectional Relationship between Sleep and Immunity against Infections. Journal of Immunology Research, 2015, 1–14. https://doi.org/10.1155/2015/678164

Ikonte, C. J., Mun, J. G., Reider, C. A., Grant, R. W., & Mitmesser, S. H. (2019). Micronutrient Inadequacy in Short Sleep: Analysis of the NHANES 2005–2016. Nutrients, 11(10), 2335. https://doi.org/10.3390/nu11102335

Imamura, M., Williams, K., Wells, M., & McGrother, C. (2015). Lifestyle interventions for the treatment of urinary incontinence in adults. Cochrane Database of Systematic Reviews. https://doi.org/10.1002/14651858.cd003505.pub5

Janeway, C. A., Travers, P., Walport, M., & Shlomchik, M. J. (2001). Immunobiology : the immune system in health and disease (5th ed.). Garland Science.

Jeczmien-Lazur, J. S., Sanetra, A. M., Pradel, K., Izowit, G., Chrobok, L., Palus-Chramiec, K., Piggins, H. D., &

Lewandowski, M. H. (2023). Metabolic cues impact non-oscillatory intergeniculate leaflet and ventral lateral geniculate nucleus: standard versus high-fat diet comparative study. The Journal of Physiology. https://doi.org/10.1113/jp283757

Jones, B. E. (2019). Arousal and sleep circuits. Neuropsychopharmacology, 45. https://doi.org/10.1038/s41386-019-0444-2

Jones, J. M. (2013, December 19). In U.S., 40% Get Less Than Recommended Amount of Sleep. Gallup.com. https://news.gallup.com/poll/166553/less-recommended-amount-sleep.aspx

Kamal Patel, M. P. H. (2022). Ornithine Research Analysis. Examine.com. https://examine.com/supplements/ornithine/

Kandel, E. R., Schwartz, J. H., Jessell, T. M., Seigelbaum, S. A., & Hudspeth, A. J. (2012). Principles of neural science (5th ed.). Mcgraw-Hill Medical.

Kareem, K. (2022, October 8). L-Ornithine : Health Benefits, Side Effects And More. Kidney Urology. https://www.kidneyurology.org/l-ornithine/

Karimi, L., Rahimi-Bashar, F., Mohammadi, S. M., Mollahadi, M., Khosh-Fetrat, M., Vahedian-Azimi, A., & Ashtari, S. (2021). The Efficacy of Eye Masks and Earplugs Interventions for Sleep Promotion in Critically Ill Patients: A Systematic Review and Meta-Analysis. Frontiers in Psychiatry, 12. https://doi.org/10.3389/

fpsyt.2021.791342

Kazemi, R., Haidarimoghadam, R., Motamedzadeh, M., Golmohamadi, R., Soltanian, A., & Zoghipaydar, M. R. (2016). Effects of Shift Work on Cognitive Performance, Sleep Quality, and Sleepiness among Petrochemical Control Room Operators. Journal of Circadian Rhythms, 14(1). https://doi.org/10.5334/jcr.134

Kim, T. W., Jeong, J.-H., & Hong, S.-C. (2015). The Impact of Sleep and Circadian Disturbance on Hormones and Metabolism. International Journal of Endocrinology, 2015, 1–9. https://doi.org/10.1155/2015/591729

Koch, C. E., Leinweber, B., Drengberg, B. C., Blaum, C., & Oster, H. (2016). Interaction between circadian rhythms and stress. Neurobiology of Stress, 6, 57–67. https://doi.org/10.1016/j.ynstr.2016.09.001

Korownyk, C., & Lindblad, A. J. (2018). Infant sleep training: rest easy?. Canadian family physician Medecin de famille canadien, 64(1), 41.

Krueger, J. M., & Opp, M. R. (2016). Sleep and Microbes. International Review of Neurobiology, 131, 207–225. https://doi.org/10.1016/bs.irn.2016.07.003

Kuhathasan, N., Dufort, A., MacKillop, J., Gottschalk, R., Minuzzi, L., & Frey, B. N. (2019). The use of cannabinoids for sleep: A critical review on clinical trials. Experimental and Clinical Psychopharmacology, 27(4), 383–401. https://doi.org/10.1037/pha0000285

Lam, C., & Chung, M.-H. (2021). Dose–response effects of light therapy on sleepiness and circadian phase shift in shift workers: a meta-analysis and moderator analysis. Scientific Reports, 11(1). https://doi.org/10.1038/s41598-021-89321-1

Lane, J. M., Vlasac, I., Anderson, S. G., Kyle, S. D., Dixon, W. G., Bechtold, D. A., Gill, S., Little, M. A., Luik, A., Loudon, A., Emsley, R., Scheer, F. A. J. L., Lawlor, D. A., Redline, S., Ray, D. W., Rutter, M. K., & Saxena, R. (2016). Genome-wide association analysis identifies novel loci for chronotype in 100,420 individuals from the UK Biobank. Nature Communications, 7(1). https://doi.org/10.1038/ncomms10889

Li, J., Vitiello, M. V., & Gooneratne, N. S. (2018). Sleep in Normal Aging. Sleep Medicine Clinics, 13(1), 1–11. https://doi.org/10.1016/j.jsmc.2017.09.001

Lindahl, T., & Barnes, D. E. (2000). Repair of Endogenous DNA Damage. Cold Spring Harbor Symposia on Quantitative Biology, 65(0), 127–134. https://doi.org/10.1101/sqb.2000.65.127

Lindberg, S. (2020, January 21). Chronotype, Sleep, and Productivity. Healthline. https://www.healthline.com/health/chronotype

Liu, P. Y., Irwin, M. R., Krueger, J. M., Gaddameedhi, S., & Van Dongen, H. P. A. (2021). Night shift schedule alters endogenous regulation of circulating cytokines. Neurobiology of Sleep and Circadian Rhythms, 10, 100063. https://doi.org/10.1016/j.nbscr.2021.100063

Lovato, N., & Lack, L. (2010). The effects of napping on cognitive functioning. Progress in Brain Research, 185, 155–166. https://doi.org/10.1016/B978-0-444-53702-7.00009-9

Luboshitzky, R., Herer, P., Levi, M., Shen-Orr, Z., & Lavie, P. (1999). Relationship between rapid eye movement sleep and testosterone secretion in normal men. Journal of andrology, 20(6), 731–737.

Luboshitzky, R., Zabari, Z., Shen-Orr, Z., Herer, P., & Lavie, P. (2001). Disruption of the Nocturnal Testosterone Rhythm by Sleep Fragmentation in Normal Men. The Journal of Clinical Endocrinology & Metabolism, 86(3), 1134–1139. https://doi.org/10.1210/jcem.86.3.7296

Ma, M. A., & Morrison, E. H. (2022). Neuroanatomy, Nucleus Suprachiasmatic. In StatPearls. StatPearls Publishing; StatPearls. https://www.ncbi.nlm.nih.gov/books/NBK546664/

Mander, B. A., Winer, J. R., & Walker, M. P. (2017). Sleep and Human Aging. Neuron, 94(1), 19–36. https://doi.org/10.1016/j.neuron.2017.02.004

Mantua, J., & Spencer, R. M. C. (2017). Exploring the nap paradox: are mid-day sleep bouts a friend or foe? Sleep Medicine, 37, 88–97. https://doi.org/10.1016/j.sleep.2017.01.019

Mattingly, S. M., Martinez, G., Young, J., Cain, M. K., & Striegel, A. (2022). Snoozing: an examination of a common method of waking. Sleep, 45(10). https://doi.org/10.1093/sleep/zsac184

McFarlane, S. J., Garcia, J. E., Verhagen, D. S., & Dyer, A. G. (2020). Alarm tones, music and their elements: Analysis of reported waking sounds to counteract sleep inertia. PLOS ONE, 15(1), e0215788. https://doi.org/10.1371/journal.pone.0215788

Medic, G., Wille, M., & Hemels, M. (2017). Short- and long-term Health Consequences of Sleep Disruption. Nature and Science of Sleep, 9(9), 151–161. https://doi.org/10.2147/nss.s134864

Miller, D. J., Sargent, C., Roach, G. D., Scanlan, A. T., Vincent, G. E., & Lastella, M. (2019). Moderate-intensity exercise performed in the evening does not impair sleep in healthy males. European Journal of Sport Science, 20(1), 80–89. https://doi.org/10.1080/17461391.2019.1611934

Mills, J. N., Minors, D. S., & Waterhouse, J. M. (1974). The circadian rhythms of human subjects without timepieces or indication of the alternation of day and night. The Journal of Physiology, 240(3), 567–594. https://doi.org/10.1113/jphysiol.1974.sp010623

Milner, C. E., & Cote, K. A. (2009). Benefits of napping in healthy adults: impact of nap length, time of day, age, and experience with napping. Journal of Sleep Research, 18(2), 272–281. https://doi.org/10.1111/j.1365-2869.2008.00718.x

Mindell, J. A., & Williamson, A. A. (2018). Benefits of a bedtime routine in young children: Sleep, development, and beyond. Sleep Medicine Reviews, 40(1), 93–108. https://doi.org/10.1016/j.smrv.2017.10.007

Mitchell, N. S., Catenacci, V. A., Wyatt, H. R., & Hill, J. O. (2011). Obesity: Overview of an Epidemic. Psychiatric Clinics of North America, 34(4), 717–732. https://doi.org/10.1016/j.psc.2011.08.005

Miyake, M., Kirisako, T., Kokubo, T., Miura, Y., Morishita, K., Okamura, H., & Tsuda, A. (2014). Randomised controlled trial of the effects of L-ornithine on stress markers and sleep quality in healthy workers. Nutrition Journal, 13(1). https://doi.org/10.1186/1475-2891-13-53

Mohd Azmi, N. A. S., Juliana, N., Azmani, S., Mohd Effendy, N., Abu, I. F., Mohd Fahmi Teng, N. I., & Das, S. (2021). Cortisol on Circadian Rhythm and Its Effect on Cardiovascular System. International Journal of Environmental Research and Public Health, 18(2), 676. https://doi.org/10.3390/ijerph18020676

Moldes, O., Dineva, D., & Ku, L. (2022). Has the COVID-19 pandemic made us more materialistic? The effect of COVID-19 and lockdown restrictions on the endorsement of materialism. Psychology & Marketing, 39(5). https://doi.org/10.1002/mar.21627

Moore, R. Y., & Card, J. P. (1994). Intergeniculate leaflet: An anatomically and functionally distinct subdivision of the lateral geniculate complex. The Journal of

Comparative Neurology, 344(3), 403–430. https://doi.org/10.1002/cne.903440306

Murillo-Rodriguez, E., Arias-Carrion, O., Sanguino-Rodriguez, K., Gonzalez-Arias, M., & Haro, R. (2009). Mechanisms of Sleep-Wake Cycle Modulation. CNS & Neurological Disorders - Drug Targets, 8(4), 245–253. https://doi.org/10.2174/187152709788921654

Nagendra, R. P., Maruthai, N., & Kutty, B. M. (2012). Meditation and Its Regulatory Role on Sleep. Frontiers in Neurology, 3. https://doi.org/10.3389/fneur.2012.00054

Nutt, D., Wilson, S., & Paterson, L. (2022). Sleep disorders as core symptoms of depression. Dialogues in Clinical Neuroscience, 10(3), 329–336. https://doi.org/10.31887/dcns.2008.10.3/dnutt

Okamoto-Mizuno, K., & Mizuno, K. (2012). Effects of thermal environment on sleep and circadian rhythm. Journal of Physiological Anthropology, 31(1). https://doi.org/10.1186/1880-6805-31-14

Okun, M. L., Mancuso, R. A., Hobel, C. J., Schetter, C. D., & Coussons-Read, M. (2018). Poor sleep quality increases symptoms of depression and anxiety in postpartum women. Journal of Behavioral Medicine, 41(5), 703–710. https://doi.org/10.1007/s10865-018-9950-7

Ong, J. C., & Smith, C. E. (2017). Using Mindfulness for the Treatment of Insomnia. Current Sleep Medicine

Reports, 3(2), 57–65. https://doi.org/10.1007/s40675-017-0068-1

Oster, H., Challet, E., Ott, V., Arvat, E., de Kloet, E. R., Dijk, D.-J., Lightman, S., Vgontzas, A., & Van Cauter, E. (2016). The functional and clinical significance of the 24-h rhythm of circulating glucocorticoids. Endocrine Reviews, 38(1), er.2015-1080. https://doi.org/10.1210/er.2015-1080

Pandi-Perumal, S. R., Zisapel, N., Srinivasan, V., & Cardinali, D. P. (2005). Melatonin and sleep in aging population. Experimental Gerontology, 40(12), 911–925. https://doi.org/10.1016/j.exger.2005.08.009

Patel, A. K., Reddy, V., Shumway, K. R., & Araujo, J. F. (2022). Physiology, Sleep Stages. In StatPearls. StatPearls Publishing; StatPearls. https://www.ncbi.nlm.nih.gov/books/NBK526132/

Peter-Derex, L., Yammine, P., Bastuji, H., & Croisile, B. (2015). Sleep and Alzheimer's disease. Sleep Medicine Reviews, 19, 29–38. https://doi.org/10.1016/j.smrv.2014.03.007

Pilorz, V., Tam, S. K. E., Hughes, S., Pothecary, C. A., Jagannath, A., Hankins, M. W., Bannerman, D. M., Lightman, S. L., Vyazovskiy, V. V., Nolan, P. M., Foster, R. G., & Peirson, S. N. (2016). Melanopsin Regulates Both Sleep-Promoting and Arousal-Promoting Responses to Light. PLoS Biology, 14(6). https://doi.org/10.1371/journal.pbio.1002482

Pinckard, K., Baskin, K. K., & Stanford, K. I. (2019). Effects of Exercise to Improve Cardiovascular Health. Frontiers in Cardiovascular Medicine, 6(69). https://doi.org/10.3389/fcvm.2019.00069

Price, A. M. H., Wake, M., Ukoumunne, O. C., & Hiscock, H. (2012). Five-Year Follow-up of Harms and Benefits of Behavioral Infant Sleep Intervention: Randomized Trial. Pediatrics, 130(4), 643–651. https://doi.org/10.1542/peds.2011-3467

Prinz, P. N., Roehrs, T. A., Vitaliano, P. P., Linnoila, M., & Weitzman, E. D. (1980). Effect of Alcohol on Sleep and Nighttime Plasma Growth Hormone and Cortisol Concentrations*. The Journal of Clinical Endocrinology & Metabolism, 51(4), 759–764. https://doi.org/10.1210/jcem-51-4-759

Purves, D., Augustine, G. J., Fitzpatrick, D., Katz, L. C., LaMantia, A.-S., McNamara, J. O., & Williams, S. M. (Eds.). (2001). Sleep and Wakefulness. In Neuroscience, 2nd edition. Sinauer Associates, Inc.

Putilov, A. A., Sveshnikov, D. S., Puchkova, A. N., Dorokhov, V. B., Bakaeva, Z. B., Yakunina, E. B., Starshinov, Y. P., Torshin, V. I., Alipov, N. N., Sergeeva, O. V., Trutneva, E. A., Lapkin, M. M., Lopatskaya, Z. N., Budkevich, R. O., Budkevich, E. V., Dyakovich, M. P., Donskaya, O. G., Plusnin, J. M., Delwiche, B., & Colomb, C. (2021). Single-Item Chronotyping (SIC), a method to self-assess diurnal types by using 6 simple charts. Personality and Individual Differences, 168, 110353. https://doi.org/10.1016/j.paid.2020.110353

Raman, S., & Coogan, A. N. (2019). Closing the Loop Between Circadian Rhythms, Sleep, and Attention Deficit Hyperactivity Disorder. Handbook of Sleep Research, 30, 707–716. https://doi.org/10.1016/b978-0-12-813743-7.00047-5

Reddy, S., Reddy, V., & Sharma, S. (2022). Physiology, Circadian Rhythm. In StatPearls. StatPearls Publishing; StatPearls. https://www.ncbi.nlm.nih.gov/books/NBK519507/

Rhodiola. (2020, October). NCCIH. https://www.nccih.nih.gov/health/rhodiola

Ribeiro, J. A., & Sebastião, A. M. (2010). Caffeine and adenosine. Journal of Alzheimer's Disease : JAD, 20 Suppl 1(20), S3-15. https://doi.org/10.3233/JAD-2010-1379

Richard, D. M., Dawes, M. A., Mathias, C. W., Acheson, A., Hill-Kapturczak, N., & Dougherty, D. M. (2009). L-Tryptophan: Basic Metabolic Functions, Behavioral Research and Therapeutic Indications. International Journal of Tryptophan Research, 2, IJTR.S2129. https://doi.org/10.4137/ijtr.s2129

Richter, D., Krämer, M. D., Tang, N. K. Y., Montgomery-Downs, H. E., & Lemola, S. (2019). Long-term effects of pregnancy and childbirth on sleep satisfaction and duration of first-time and experienced mothers and fathers. Sleep, 42(4). https://doi.org/10.1093/sleep/zsz015

Rijo-Ferreira, F., & Takahashi, J. S. (2019). Genomics of circadian rhythms in health and disease. Genome Medicine, 11(1). https://doi.org/10.1186/s13073-019-0704-0

Roddick, J., & Cherney, K. (2020, July 28). Sleep Disorders: Causes, Diagnosis & Treatments (C. Clark & R. Dasgupta, Eds.). Healthline. https://www.healthline.com/health/sleep/disorders

Roenneberg, T. (2015). Having Trouble Typing? What on Earth Is Chronotype? Journal of Biological Rhythms, 30(6), 487–491. https://doi.org/10.1177/0748730415603835

Romdhani, M., Souissi, N., Dergaa, I., Moussa-Chamari, I., Abene, O., Chtourou, H., Sahnoun, Z., Driss, T., Chamari, K., & Hammouda, O. (2021). The Effect of Experimental Recuperative and Appetitive Post-lunch Nap Opportunities, With or Without Caffeine, on Mood and Reaction Time in Highly Trained Athletes. Frontiers in Psychology, 12. https://doi.org/10.3389/fpsyg.2021.720493

Rosekind, M. R., Smith, R. M., Miller, D. L., Co, E. L., Gregory, K. B., Webbon, L. L., Gander, P. H., & Lebacqz, J. V. (1995). Alertness management: strategic naps in operational settings. Journal of Sleep Research, 4, 62–66. https://doi.org/10.1111/j.1365-2869.1995.tb00229.x

Roser, M. (2016, December 23). Proof that life is getting better for humanity, in 5 charts. Vox. https://

www.vox.com/the-big-idea/2016/12/23/14062168/
history-global-conditions-charts-life-span-poverty

Rundo, J. V., & Downey, R. (2019). Polysomnography.
Handbook of Clinical Neurology, 160, 381–392. https://
doi.org/10.1016/B978-0-444-64032-1.00025-4

Sack, R. L., Auckley, D., Auger, R. R., Carskadon, M. A.,
Wright, K. P., Vitiello, M. V., & Zhdanova, I. V. (2007).
Circadian Rhythm Sleep Disorders: Part II, Advanced
Sleep Phase Disorder, Delayed Sleep Phase Disorder,
Free-Running Disorder, and Irregular Sleep-Wake
Rhythm. Sleep, 30(11), 1484–1501. https://doi.org/
10.1093/sleep/30.11.1484

Sack, R. L., Auckley, D., Auger, R. R., Carskadon, M. A.,
Wright, K. P., Vitiello, M. V., Zhdanova, I. V., & American
Academy of Sleep Medicine. (2007). Circadian rhythm
sleep disorders: part I, basic principles, shift work and
jet lag disorders. An American Academy of Sleep
Medicine review. Sleep, 30(11), 1460–1483. https://
doi.org/10.1093/sleep/30.11.1460

Sateia, M. J. (2009). Update on Sleep and Psychiatric
Disorders. Chest, 135(5), 1370–1379. https://doi.org/
10.1378/chest.08-1834

Scullin, M. K., Krueger, M. L., Ballard, H. K., Pruett, N., &
Bliwise, D. L. (2018). The effects of bedtime writing on
difficulty falling asleep: A polysomnographic study
comparing to-do lists and completed activity lists.
Journal of Experimental Psychology: General, 147(1),
139–146. https://doi.org/10.1037/xge0000374

Seladi-Schulman, J. (2021, February 1). Elevating Legs: Health Benefits, How To, Precautions. Healthline. https://www.healthline.com/health/elevating-legs

Shafiee, M. A., Charest, A. F., Cheema-Dhadli, S., Glick, D. N., Napolova, O., Roozbeh, J., Semenova, E., Sharman, A., & Halperin, M. L. (2005). Defining conditions that lead to the retention of water: The importance of the arterial sodium concentration. Kidney International, 67(2), 613–621. https://doi.org/10.1111/j.1523-1755.2005.67117.x

Sharpe, E., Lacombe, A., Butler, M. P., Hanes, D., & Bradley, R. (2020). A Closer Look at Yoga Nidra: Sleep Lab Protocol. International Journal of Yoga Therapy. https://doi.org/10.17761/2021-d-20-00004

Siegel, J. M. (2005). Clues to the functions of mammalian sleep. Nature, 437(7063), 1264–1271. https://doi.org/10.1038/nature04285

Singh, N., Bhalla, M., De Jager, P., & Gilca, M. (2011). An Overview on Ashwagandha: A Rasayana (Rejuvenator) of Ayurveda. African Journal of Traditional, Complementary and Alternative Medicines, 8(5S). https://doi.org/10.4314/ajtcam.v8i5s.9

Smith, A., Conger, J., Hedayati, B., Kim, J., Amoozadeh, S., & Mehta, M. (2020). The effect of a screen protector on blue light intensity emitted from different hand-held devices. Middle East African Journal of Ophthalmology, 27(3), 177. https://doi.org/10.4103/meajo.meajo_2_20

Souissi, M., Chtourou, H., Zrane, A., Cheikh, R. B., Dogui, M., Tabka, Z., & Souissi, N. (2012). Effect of time-of-day of aerobic maximal exercise on the sleep quality of trained subjects. Biological Rhythm Research, 43(3), 323–330. https://doi.org/10.1080/09291016.2011.589159

St-Onge, M.-P., Mikic, A., & Pietrolungo, C. E. (2016). Effects of Diet on Sleep Quality. Advances in Nutrition, 7(5), 938–949. https://doi.org/10.3945/an.116.012336

St-Onge, M.-P., Roberts, A., Shechter, A., & Choudhury, A. R. (2016). Fiber and Saturated Fat Are Associated with Sleep Arousals and Slow Wave Sleep. Journal of Clinical Sleep Medicine, 12(01), 19–24. https://doi.org/10.5664/jcsm.5384

Sukumaran, S., Almon, R. R., DuBois, D. C., & Jusko, W. J. (2010). Circadian rhythms in gene expression: Relationship to physiology, disease, drug disposition and drug action☆. Advanced Drug Delivery Reviews, 62(9-10), 904–917. https://doi.org/10.1016/j.addr.2010.05.009

Szymusiak, R. (2018). Body temperature and sleep. Handbook of Clinical Neurology, 156, 341–351. https://doi.org/10.1016/b978-0-444-63912-7.00020-5

Takakura, M., Nagamachi, S., Nishigawa, T., Takahashi, Y., & Furuse, M. (2022). Supplementation of L-Ornithine Could Increase Sleep-like Behavior in the Mouse Pups. Metabolites, 12(12), 1241. https://doi.org/10.3390/metabo12121241

Tassi, P., & Muzet, A. (2000). Sleep inertia. Sleep Medicine Reviews, 4(4), 341–353. https://doi.org/10.1053/smrv.2000.0098

te Kulve, M., Schlangen, L. J. M., & van Marken Lichtenbelt, W. D. (2019). Early evening light mitigates sleep compromising physiological and alerting responses to subsequent late evening light. Scientific Reports, 9(1). https://doi.org/10.1038/s41598-019-52352-w

Tempaku, P. F., Mazzotti, D. R., & Tufik, S. (2015). Telomere length as a marker of sleep loss and sleep disturbances: a potential link between sleep and cellular senescence. Sleep Medicine, 16(5), 559–563. https://doi.org/10.1016/j.sleep.2015.02.519

Toppila, J., Asikainen, M., Alanko, L., Turek, F., Stenberg, D., & Porkka-Heiskanen, T. (1996). The effect of REM sleep deprivation on somatostatin and growth hormone-releasing hormone gene expression in the rat hypothalamus. Journal of Sleep Research, 5(2), 115–122. https://doi.org/10.1046/j.1365-2869.1996.d01-66.x

Tosini, G., Ferguson, I., & Tsubota, K. (2016). Effects of blue light on the circadian system and eye physiology. Molecular Vision, 22, 61-72. https://www.ncbi.nlm.nih.gov/pmc/articles/PMC4734149/

Triantafillou, S., Saeb, S., Lattie, E. G., Mohr, D. C., & Kording, K. P. (2019). Relationship Between Sleep Quality and Mood: Ecological Momentary Assessment Study. JMIR Mental Health, 6(3), e12613. https://

doi.org/10.2196/12613

Trotti, L. M. (2017). Waking up is the hardest thing I do all day: Sleep inertia and sleep drunkenness. Sleep Medicine Reviews, 35, 76–84. https://doi.org/10.1016/j.smrv.2016.08.005

Tyagi, V., Scordo, M., Yoon, R. S., Liporace, F. A., & Greene, L. W. (2017). Revisiting the role of testosterone: Are we missing something? Reviews in Urology, 19(1), 16–24.

University of Chicago Library. (2016). Mammoth Cave - Discovering the Beauty and Charm of the Wilderness - The University of Chicago Library. https://www.lib.uchicago.edu/collex/exhibits/discovering-beauty/mammoth-cave/

Uriu, K., & Tei, H. (2019). A saturated reaction in repressor synthesis creates a daytime dead zone in circadian clocks. PLOS Computational Biology, 15(2), e1006787. https://doi.org/10.1371/journal.pcbi.1006787

Urry, L. A., Cain, M. L., Wasserman, S. A., Minorsky, P. V., Orr, R. B., Campbell, N. A., & Reece, J. (2020). Campbell biology (12th ed.). Pearson.

Van Cauter, E., & Plat, L. (1996). Physiology of growth hormone secretion during sleep. The Journal of Pediatrics, 128(5), S32–S37. https://doi.org/10.1016/s0022-3476(96)70008-2

Vandekerckhove, M., & Wang, Y. (2017). Emotion, emotion regulation and sleep: An intimate relationship. AIMS Neuroscience, 5(1), 1–17. https://doi.org/10.3934/Neuroscience.2018.1.1

Vitale, J. A., & Weydahl, A. (2017). Chronotype, Physical Activity, and Sport Performance: A Systematic Review. Sports Medicine, 47(9), 1859–1868. https://doi.org/10.1007/s40279-017-0741-z

Wahl, S., Engelhardt, M., Schaupp, P., Lappe, C., & Ivanov, I. V. (2019). The inner clock—Blue light sets the human rhythm. Journal of Biophotonics, 12(12). https://doi.org/10.1002/jbio.201900102

Waterhouse, J., Reilly, T., & Edwards, B. (2004). The stress of travel. Journal of Sports Sciences, 22(10), 946–966. https://doi.org/10.1080/02640410400000264

Wehrens, S. M. T., Christou, S., Isherwood, C., Middleton, B., Gibbs, M. A., Archer, S. N., Skene, D. J., & Johnston, J. D. (2017). Meal Timing Regulates the Human Circadian System. Current Biology : CB, 27(12), 1768-1775.e3. https://doi.org/10.1016/j.cub.2017.04.059

Wickwire, E. M., Geiger-Brown, J., Scharf, S. M., & Drake, C. L. (2017). Shift Work and Shift Work Sleep Disorder. Chest, 151(5), 1156–1172. https://doi.org/10.1016/j.chest.2016.12.007

Wielek, T., Del Giudice, R., Lang, A., Wislowska, M., Ott, P., & Schabus, M. (2019). On the development of sleep states in the first weeks of life. PLOS ONE, 14(10), e0224521. https://doi.org/10.1371/journal.pone.0224521

Wiginton, K. (2021, July 27). Cannabis, CBD, and Sleep. WebMD. https://www.webmd.com/sleep-disorders/features/cannabis-cbd-sleep

Woelders, T., Wams, E. J., Gordijn, M. C. M., Beersma, D. G. M., & Hut, R. A. (2018). Integration of color and intensity increases time signal stability for the human circadian system when sunlight is obscured by clouds. Scientific Reports, 8(1). https://doi.org/10.1038/s41598-018-33606-5

Wong, B. J., & Hollowed, C. G. (2016). Current concepts of active vasodilation in human skin. Temperature: Multidisciplinary Biomedical Journal, 4(1), 41–59. https://doi.org/10.1080/23328940.2016.1200203

World Health Organisation. (2022, October 5). Physical activity. Physical Activity; World Health Organization. https://www.who.int/news-room/fact-sheets/detail/physical-activity

Wright, K. P., Hull, J. T., & Czeisler, C. A. (2002). Relationship between alertness, performance, and body temperature in humans. American Journal of Physiology. Regulatory, Integrative and Comparative Physiology, 283(6), R1370-7. https://doi.org/10.1152/ajpregu.00205.2002

Yetman, D. (2021, January 11). Polyphasic Sleep:

Potential Benefits, Risks, If You Should Try It. Healthline. https://www.healthline.com/health/polyphasic-sleep

Zee, P. C., Attarian, H., & Videnovic, A. (2013). Circadian Rhythm Abnormalities. Continuum: Lifelong Learning in Neurology, 19(1), 132–147. https://doi.org/10.1212/01.con.0000427209.21177.aa

Zhu, Y., Liu, X., Ding, X., Wang, F., & Geng, X. (2018). Telomere and its role in the aging pathways: telomere shortening, cell senescence and mitochondria dysfunction. Biogerontology, 20(1), 1–16. https://doi.org/10.1007/s10522-018-9769-1

Zisapel, N. (2018). New perspectives on the role of melatonin in human sleep, circadian rhythms and their regulation. British Journal of Pharmacology, 175(16), 3190–3199. https://doi.org/10.1111/bph.14116

Made in United States
Troutdale, OR
04/05/2024

18936115R00094